Waldenström Macroglobulinemia

Editors

JORGE J. CASTILLO
SHAYNA SAROSIEK
PRASHANT KAPOOR

HEMATOLOGY/ONCOLOGY CLINICS OF NORTH AMERICA

www.hemonc.theclinics.com

Consulting Editors
GEORGE P. CANELLOS
EDWARD J. BENZ JR.

August 2023 • Volume 37 • Number 4

ELSEVIER

1600 John F. Kennedy Boulevard • Suite 1800 • Philadelphia, Pennsylvania, 19103-2899

http://www.theclinics.com

HEMATOLOGY/ONCOLOGY CLINICS OF NORTH AMERICA Volume 37, Number 4
August 2023 ISSN 0889-8588, ISBN 13: 978-0-443-18298-3

Editor: Stacy Eastman
Developmental Editor: Ann Gielou M. Posedio

Hematology/Oncology Clinics (ISSN 0889-8588) is published bimonthly by Elsevier Inc., 360 Park Avenue South, New York, NY 10010-1710. Months of issue are February, April, June, August, October, and December. Business and Editorial Offices: 1600 John F. Kennedy Blvd., Ste. 1800, Philadelphia, PA 19103–2899. Customer Service Office: 3251 Riverport Lane, Maryland Heights, MO 63043. Periodicals postage paid at New York, NY and at additional mailing offices. Subscription prices are $470.00 per year (domestic individuals), $1190.00 per year (domestic institutions), $100.00 per year (domestic students/residents), $495.00 per year (Canadian individuals), $100.00 per year (Canadian students/residents), $1232.00 per year (Canadian institutions) $563.00 per year (international individuals), $1232.00 per year (international institutions), and $255.00 per year (international students/residents). International air speed delivery is included in all *Clinics* subscription prices. All prices are subject to change without notice. **POSTMASTER:** Send address changes to *Hematology/Oncology Clinics of North America*, Elsevier Health Sciences Division, Subscription Customer Service, 3251 Riverport Lane, Maryland Heights, MO 63043. Customer Service (orders, claims, online, change of address): Elsevier Health Sciences Division, Subscription **Customer Service, 3251 Riverport Lane, Maryland Heights, MO 63043. Tel: 1-800-654-2452 (U.S. and Canada); 314-447-8871 (outside U.S. and Canada). Fax: 314-447-8029. E-mail: journalscustomerservice-usa@elsevier.com (for print support); journalsonlinesupport-usa@elsevier.com (for online support).**

Reprints. For copies of 100 or more, of articles in this publication, please contact the Commercial Reprints Department, Elsevier Inc., 360 Park Avenue South, New York, New York 10010-1710; Tel.: 212-633-3874, Fax: 212-633-3820, E-mail: reprints@elsevier.com.

Hematology/Oncology Clinics of North America is covered in *MEDLINE/PubMed (Index Medicus), EMBASE/ Excerpta Medica, and BIOSIS.*

Contributors

CONSULTING EDITORS

GEORGE P. CANELLOS, MD
William Rosenberg Professor of Medicine, Department of Medical Oncology, Dana-Farber Cancer Institute, Boston, Massachusetts, USA

EDWARD J. BENZ Jr, MD
President and CEO Emeritus, Dana-Farber Cancer Institute, Director Emeritus, Dana-Farber/Harvard Cancer Center, Richard and Susan Smith Distinguished Professor of Medicine, Professor of Pediatrics, Professor of Genetics, Harvard Medical School, Boston, Massachusetts, USA

EDITORS

JORGE J. CASTILLO, MD
Bing Center for Waldenström Macroglobulinemia, Dana-Farber Cancer Institute, Associate Professor, Harvard Medical School, Boston, Massachusetts, USA

SHAYNA SAROSIEK, MD
Bing Center for Waldenström Macroglobulinemia, Dana-Farber Cancer Institute, Department of Medicine, Harvard Medical School, Boston, Massachusetts, USA

PRASHANT KAPOOR, MD, FACP
Associate Professor of Medicine, Division of Hematology, Department of Internal Medicine, Mayo Clinic, Rochester, Minnesota, USA

AUTHORS

JITHMA P. ABEYKOON, MD
Division of Hematology, Mayo Clinic, Rochester, Minnesota, USA

CHRISTIAN BUSKE, MD
University Hospital Ulm, Institute for Experimental Cancer Research, Ulm, Germany

JORGE J. CASTILLO, MD
Bing Center for Waldenström Macroglobulinemia, Dana-Farber Cancer Institute, Associate Professor, Harvard Medical School, Boston, Massachusetts, USA

CARLOS CHIATTONE, MD
Hematology and Oncology Discipline, Santa Casa Medical School, Sao Paulo, Brazil

SHIRLEY D'SA, FRCP, FRCPath, MD(Res)
Consultant Haematologist, Department of Haematology, Centre for Waldenströms Macroglobulinaemia and Related Conditions, University College London Hospitals NHS Foundation Trust, London, United Kingdom

ALAIN DELMER, MD
Department of Hematology, University Hospital of Reims and UFR Médecine, Reims, France

MELETIOS A. DIMOPOULOS, MD
Department of Clinical Therapeutics, National and Kapodistrian University of Athens, Athens, Greece

ERIC DUROT, MD
Department of Hematology, University Hospital of Reims and UFR Médecine, Reims, France

CARLOS FERNÁNDEZ DE LARREA, MD, PhD
Department of Hematology, Amyloidosis and Myeloma Unit, Hospital Clínic de Barcelona, Institut D'Investigacions Biomèdiques August Pi I Sunyer, University of Barcelona, Barcelona, Spain

RAMÓN GARCÍA-SANZ, MD, PhD
Department of Hematology, University Hospital of Salamanca, Research Biomedical Institute of Salamanca (IBSAL), Accelerator Project, Centro de Investigación Biomédica en Red-Cáncer (CIBERONC) CB16/12/00369 and Center for Cancer Research-IBMCC (USAL-CSIC), Salamanca, Spain

PRASHANT KAPOOR, MD, FACP
Associate Professor of Medicine, Division of Hematology, Department of Internal Medicine, Mayo Clinic, Rochester, Minnesota, USA

EFSTATHIOS KASTRITIS, MD
Department of Clinical Therapeutics, National and Kapodistrian University of Athens, Athens, Greece

VERONIQUE LEBLOND, MD, PhD
Consultant Haematologist, Department of Haematology, Sorbonne University and Pitié Salpêtrière Hospital, Paris, France

MICHAEL P. LUNN, FRCP, PhD
Consultant Neurologist and Joint Co-Ed Cochrane Neuromuscular, National Hospital for Neurology and Neurosurgery, London, United Kingdom

HUMBERTO MARTÍNEZ-CORDERO, MD, MSc
Instituto Nacional de Cancerología, Bogotá, Colombia

JEFFREY V. MATOUS, MD
Colorado Blood Cancer Institute, Sarah Cannon Research Institute, Denver, Colorado, USA

MONIQUE C. MINNEMA, MD, PhD
Professor, Department of Hematology, Internist-Hematologist, UMC Utrecht, Utrecht, the Netherlands

PIERRE MOREL, MD
Professor, Department of Hematology, University Hospital of Amiens, Amiens, France

DAVID F. MORENO, MD
Department of Hematology, Amyloidosis and Myeloma Unit, Hospital Clínic de Barcelona, Institut D'Investigacions Biomèdiques August Pi I Sunyer, University of Barcelona, Barcelona, Spain

MARIA LIA PALOMBA, MD
Memorial Sloan Kettering Cancer Center, New York, New York, USA

JONAS PALUDO, MD
Division of Hematology, Mayo Clinic, Rochester, Minnesota, USA

ELOISA RIVA, MD
Clinical Hospital Dr Manuel Quintela, University of the Republic, British Hospital, Montevideo, Uruguay

SHAYNA SAROSIEK, MD
Bing Center for Waldenström Macroglobulinemia, Dana-Farber Cancer Institute, Department of Medicine, Harvard Medical School, Boston, Massachusetts, USA

SARAH J. SCHEP, MD, PhD
Department of Hematology, Internist-Hematologist, HAGA Ziekenhuis, The Hague, the Netherlands

EIRINI SOLIA, MD
Department of Clinical Therapeutics, National and Kapodistrian University of Athens, Athens, Greece

DIPTI TALAULIKAR, PhD, FRCPA, FRACP
Professor, Department of Hematology, Canberra Health Services, College of Health and Medicine, Australian National University, Canberra, Australian Capital Territory, Australia

ALESSANDRA TEDESCHI, MD
Department of Hematology, Niguarda Cancer Center, ASST Grande Ospedale Metropolitano Niguarda, Milano, Italy

VANIA TIETSCHE DE MORAES HUNGRÍA, MD
Irmandade Da Santa Casa De Misericordia De São Paulo, Sao Paulo, Brazil

OLIVER TOMKINS, BMBS, MRCP
Haematology Fellow, Department of Haematology, Centre for Waldenströms Macroglobulinaemia and Related Conditions, University College London Hospitals NHS Foundation Trust, London, United Kingdom

CÉCILE TOMOWIAK, MD
Hematology Department and Centre d'Investigations Cliniques (CIC) 1082 INSERM, University Hospital, Poitiers, France

ELISE TOUSSAINT, MD
Department of Hematology, Institut de Cancérologie Strasbourg Europe (ICANS), Strasbourg, France

MARZIA VARETTONI, MD
Division of Hematology, Fondazione IRCCS Policlinico San Matteo, Pavia, Italy

KARINE VIALA, MD
Consultant Neurologist, Department of Clinical Neurophysiology, Sorbonne University and Pitié Salpêtrière Hospital, Paris, France

JOSEPHINE M.I. VOS, MD, PhD
Department of Hematology, Internist-Hematologist, Amsterdam UMC, University of Amsterdam, LYMMCARE, Cancer Center Amsterdam, Amsterdam, the Netherlands

DAMIEN ROOS-WEIL, MD, PhD
Consultant Haematologist, Department of Haematology, Sorbonne University and Pitié Salpêtrière Hospital, Paris, France

Contents

With the increasing availability of sequencing techniques and new polymerase chain reaction-based methods, data regarding the genomic profile of Waldenström macroglobulinemia (WM) are being continuously analyzed and reproduced. *MYD88* and *CXCR4* mutations are highly prevalent in all the stages of WM, including the early IgM monoclonal gammopathy of undetermined significance or a more advanced stage, such as smoldering WM. Thus, there is a need to define genotypes before starting either standard treatment regimens or clinical trials. Here, we review the genomic profile of WM and its clinical implications while focusing on recent advances.

Despite the introduction of effective novel agents, chemoimmunotherapy (CIT), with its widespread use, retains relevance and is one of the 2 vastly disparate strategies to treat Waldenström macroglobulinemia (WM), the alternative being the Bruton tyrosine kinase inhibitor (BTKi)-based approach. Considerable evidence over the past decades supports the integration of the monoclonal anti-CD20 antibody, rituximab, to the CIT backbone in WM, a CD20+ malignancy. Besides substantial efficacy, the finite duration of the treatment, coupled with lower rates of cumulative and long-term, clinically significant adverse effects and greater affordability, make CIT appealing, notwithstanding the lack of quality-of-life data with such an approach in WM. A phase 3 randomized controlled trial reported substantially higher efficacy and a more favorable safety profile of the bendamustine-rituximab (BR) doublet compared with R-CHOP (rituximab, cyclophosphamide, doxorubicin, vincristine, and prednisone) among patients with WM. Subsequent studies reaffirmed its high efficacy and tolerability, making BR the mainstay of managing treatment-naïve patients with WM. High-quality evidence supporting the use of BR over Dexamethasone, Rituximab, and Cyclophosphamide (DRC), another commonly used regimen, is lacking, as is its comparison with the continuous BTKi-based approach. However, DRC appeared less potent than BR in cross-trial comparisons and retrospective series involving treatment-naïve patients with WM. Additionally, a recent retrospective, international study demonstrated comparable outcomes with fixed-duration BR and continuous ibrutinib monotherapy among previously untreated, age-matched patients exhibiting *MYD88*^{L265P} mutation. However, unlike ibrutinib, BR appears effective irrespective of the *MYD88* mutation status. CIT, preferably BR, is well suited to serve as the control arm (comparator) regimen against which novel targeted agents may be evaluated as frontline therapies for WM in high-quality trials. Purine analog-based CIT has been extensively evaluated in WM, although its use has waned, even in the multiply relapsed patient population, as effective and safer alternatives emerge.

Proteasome inhibitors (PIs) have long been used in myeloma therapy but also for Waldenström macroglobulinemia. Their use has been successful and has also been investigated for the frontline management of the disease. Bortezomib was effective either as a single agent or in combination with other regimens with high response rates observed in most studies, despite its adverse effects, especially neurotoxicity, which remains a major concern. Clinical trials with second-generation PIs such as carfilzomib and ixazomib have also been conducted, always in combination with immunotherapy in previously untreated patients. They have been shown to be active and neuropathy-sparing treatment options.

The discovery of MYD88 (L265P) mutation led to investigating BTK inhibitors in Waldenström macroglobulinemia (WM). Ibrutinib, the first-in-class agent, was approved based on a phase II trial in relapsed/refractory patients. In the phase III iNNOVATE study, the combination of rituximab and ibrutinib was compared with rituximab and placebo in treatment-naïve and relapsed/refractory patients. Second-generation BTK inhibitor, zanubrutinib, was compared with Ibrutinib in MYD88-mutated WM patients in the phase III ASPEN trial, whereas acalabrutinib was investigated in a phase II trial. Here, we discuss the role of BTK inhibitors in treatment-naïve patients with WM based on currently available evidence.

Despite substantial progress in the clinical management of Waldenström's Macroglobulinemia (WM) and the emergence of chemotherapy-free approaches such as BTK inhibitors, WM is still a disease in which current treatments fail to cure and are in part associated with significant toxicities, compromising treatment outcome and quality of life. Thus, the vision for future front-line therapy should be to develop regimens which combine improved efficacy and excellent applicability with a low toxicity profile. Conventional immunochemotherapy such as bendamustine-rituximab is highly active but limited by hematotoxicity and long-lasting immunosuppression. Thus, further intensification of this treatment concept will most likely not be successful. Chemotherapy-free approaches such as BTK inhibitors have already changed the treatment landscape in WM, but still have major limitations such as the need for non-fixed duration treatment. Most probably, the combination of non-chemotherapy based, targeted approaches with different modes of action will ensure that we at least come closer to our vision of achieving functional cure in WM in the near future.

Ramón García-Sanz and Alessandra Tedeschi

Waldenström's macroglobulinemia (WM) is an immunoglobulin M monoclonal gammopathy produced by a bone marrow lymphoplasmacytic lymphoma, an indolent non-Hodgkin lymphoma in which the cure is still an unmet challenge. Combinations with alkylating agents, purine analogs, and monoclonal antibodies, Bruton tyrosine kinase, and proteasome inhibitors are used for the treatment of relapsed and refractory patients. Moreover, new additional agents can be seen on the horizon as potential effective therapies. No consensus on a preferred treatment in the relapsed setting is available yet.

Shayna Sarosiek and Jorge J. Castillo

Owing to the indolent nature of Waldenström macroglobulinemia, most patients experience a prolonged life expectancy, although many lines of therapy will likely be required to maintain disease control. Despite the currently available therapies, most patients will develop intolerance or resistance to multiple treatments. Therefore, new therapeutic options are being developed with a focus on targeted agents, such as novel Bruton tyrosine kinase (BTK) inhibitors and BTK degraders, as well as C-X-C chemokine receptor type 4, mucosa-associated lymphoid tissue translocation protein 1, and interleukin-1 receptor-associated kinase 4.

Oliver Tomkins, Veronique Leblond, Michael P. Lunn, Karine Viala, Damien Roos-Weil, and Shirley D'Sa

The immunoglobulin M (IgM)-associated peripheral neuropathies (PN) are a heterogeneous group of disorders representing most paraproteinemic neuropathy cases. They are associated with IgM monoclonal gammopathy of undetermined significance (MGUS) or Waldenström macroglobulinemia. Establishing a causal link between a paraprotein and neuropathy can be challenging but is necessary to adopt an appropriate therapeutic approach. The most common type of IgM-PN is anti-myelin-associated-glycoprotein neuropathy, but half of the cases are of other causes. Progressive functional impairment is an indication for treatment, even when the underlying disorder is IgM MGUS, involving either rituximab monotherapy or combination chemotherapy to achieve clinical stabilization.

Sarah J. Schep, Josephine M.I. Vos, and Monique C. Minnema

Bing–Neel syndrome is a rare manifestation of Waldenström macroglobulinemia (WM), which is caused by infiltration of the malignant lymphoplasmacytic cells in the central nervous system. Patients can present with a diverse range of neurologic symptoms, and differentiation with other comorbidities seen in WM, such as immunoglobulin M-related polyneuropathy, can be challenging. Both the rarity of this disorder and the heterogeneity of the clinical presentation often cause a significant diagnostic delay with the risk of permanent neurologic damage. This review summarizes current knowledge regarding diagnosis, treatment and prognosis of Bing-Neel syndrome.

Dipti Talaulikar, Cécile Tomowiak, Elise Toussaint, Pierre Morel,
Prashant Kapoor, Jorge J. Castillo, Alain Delmer, and Eric Durot

Histologic transformation (HT) to diffuse large B-cell lymphoma occurs rarely in Waldenström macroglobulinemia, with higher incidence in *MYD88* wild-type patients. HT is suspected clinically when rapidly enlarging lymph nodes, elevated lactate dehydrogenase levels, or extranodal disease occur. Histologic assessment is required for diagnosis. HT carries a worse prognosis compared with nontransformed Waldenström macroglobulinemia. A validated prognostic score based on three adverse risk factors stratifies three risk groups. The most common frontline treatment is chemoimmunotherapy, such as R-CHOP. Central nervous system prophylaxis should be considered if feasible and consolidation with autologous transplant should be discussed in fit patients responding to chemoimmunotherapy.

Eloisa Riva, Vania Tietsche de Moraes Hungría, Carlos Chiattone, and
Humberto Martínez-Cordero

Waldenström macroglobulinemia (WM) is a rare, indolent, and currently incurable B-cell neoplasm characterized by monoclonal immunoglobulin M gammopathy, frequent nodal involvement, and lymphoplasmacytic infiltration of the bone marrow. The clinical pattern at diagnosis is similar to that reported in developed countries but, unfortunately, the tools for a complete diagnosis and access to novel therapies are suboptimal. Older drugs such as bendamustine, cyclophosphamide, and chlorambucil may still play a role in treating WM. Prospective studies in resource-limited regions are required to further evaluate these essential aspects of the disease. In this document, we issue recommendations based on our local reality.

HEMATOLOGY/ONCOLOGY CLINICS OF NORTH AMERICA

SERIES OF RELATED INTEREST

Surgical Oncology Clinics
https://www.surgonc.theclinics.com/
Advances in Oncology
https://www.advances-oncology.com/

THE CLINICS ARE AVAILABLE ONLINE!
Access your subscription at:
www.theclinics.com

Preface

Waldenström Macroglobulinemia: A Myriad of Effective Treatment Options, but Still Work to be Done

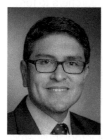
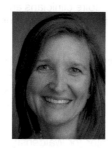
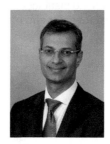

Jorge J. Castillo, MD   Shayna Sarosiek, MD   Prashant Kapoor, MD

Editors

There have been numerous advances in treating patients with Waldenström macroglobulinemia (WM) in recent years. Since 2015, the US Food and Drug Administration and the European Medicines Agency have approved the Bruton tyrosine kinase (BTK) inhibitors, ibrutinib, with or without rituximab, and zanubrutinib for treatment-naïve and previously treated patients with WM. In addition, with new compelling evidence, the National Comprehensive Cancer Network has endorsed using the novel proteasome inhibitors, ixazomib and carfilzomib (combined with dexamethasone and rituximab), the BTK inhibitor acalabrutinib, and the BCL2 antagonist, venetoclax. In the present issue of the *Hematology/Oncology Clinics of North America*, we bring together an amazing team of clinician-scientists to delve into the most significant advances with direct clinical impact in managing patients with WM.

Drs Moreno and Fernandez de Larrea discuss the clinical implications of *MYD88* and *CXCR4* mutations (among others) in treating WM. Dr Bustoros provides precious insights into managing patients with smoldering WM, focusing on a novel scoring system for patients with asymptomatic WM. Dr Kapoor and colleagues support the frontline management of WM with chemoimmunotherapy, given its high efficacy. Dr Kastritis and colleagues review the use of proteasome inhibitors in managing treatment-naïve patients with WM. Drs Varettoni and Matous provide the data supporting covalent BTK inhibitors in WM, arguably the most active oral agents to treat WM. Drs Buske and Palomba look into the future of frontline clinical trials in WM. Drs Garcia-Sanz and Tedeschi delve into managing previously treated patients with WM, an area of increased research interest. Drs Sarosiek and Castillo focus on agents

Hematol Oncol Clin N Am 37 (2023) xiii–xiv
https://doi.org/10.1016/j.hoc.2023.04.021
0889-8588/23/© 2023 Published by Elsevier Inc.

hemonc.theclinics.com

with novel mechanisms of action undergoing clinical development in WM. Dr D'Sa and colleagues review the complexities of evaluating and treating patients with often debilitating IgM-related peripheral neuropathies. Dr Minnema and colleagues discuss the nuances of managing patients with Bing-Neel syndrome, a rare neurologic syndrome with unique diagnostic and therapeutic challenges. Dr Durot and colleagues review the existing data on managing aggressive histologic transformation in WM, an infrequent complication associated with high morbidity and mortality. Finally, Dr Riva and colleagues describe the challenge of treating patients with WM in limited-resource settings.

With this issue, we hope not only to inform practitioners of the emerging data supporting the different treatment options in WM, which continue to expand, but also to foster collaboration among institutions and inspire clinicians and researchers to forge ahead with their quest for safer and more effective therapies for WM.

Jorge J. Castillo, MD
Bing Center for Waldenström Macroglobulinemia
Dana-Farber Cancer Institute
450 Brookline Avenue
Boston, MA 02115, USA

Shayna Sarosiek, MD
Bing Center for Waldenström Macroglobulinemia
Dana-Farber Cancer Institute
450 Brookline Avenue
Boston, MA 02115, USA

Prashant Kapoor, MD
Division of Hematology
Mayo Clinic
200 First Street SW
Rochester, MN 55905, USA

E-mail addresses:
jorgej_castillo@dfci.harvard.edu (J.J. Castillo)
shayna_sarosiek@dfci.harvard.edu (S. Sarosiek)
kapoor.prashant@mayo.edu (P. Kapoor)

Clinical Implications of Genomic Profile in Waldenström Macroglobulinemia

David F. Moreno, MD[a,b,*],
Carlos Fernández de Larrea, MD, PhD[a,b,**]

KEYWORDS

- Genomics • Waldenström • Clinical impact

KEY POINTS

- MYD88 L265P is the most prevalent somatic mutation in Waldenström macroglobulinemia (more than 90%), followed by CXCR4 nonsense mutations (up to 40%).
- MYD88 and CXCR4 mutations delineate clinical phenotypes in patients with Waldenström macroglobulinemia; thus, improving the diagnosis and treatment.
- Droplet digital polymerase chain reaction is a promising tool to identify and quantify precisely the MYD88 L265P and nonsense CXCR4 mutations, even in earlier stages of the disease.

INTRODUCTION

Waldenström macroglobulinemia (WM) is characterized by highly recurrent somatic mutations in the myeloid differentiation factor 88 (*MYD88*) and the C-X-C motif chemokine receptor 4 (*CXCR4*) genes.[1,2] More than 90% of patients with WM harbor *MYD88* mutations, whereas *CXCR4* mutations account for up to 40%.[3] A change from leucine to proline at position 265 in *MYD88*, also known as *MYD88* L265P, accounts for almost all mutations identified in that gene.[2] However, a wide spectrum of nonsense and frameshift mutations in *CXCR4* has been reported. However, the most prevalent are those found at position 338, causing a stop codon (*CXCR4* S338*).[1] Presymptomatic stages such as IgM monoclonal gammopathy of undetermined significance (MGUS) or smoldering WM (SWM) also show a similar profile.[4,5] Various reports have described the 3 most common genotypes in WM: *MYD88* mutated (mut) *CXCR4* wild type (wt), *MYD88*mut *CXCR4*mut, and *MYD88*wt *CXCR4*wt.[6] With the advent of new sequencing

[a] Department of Hematology, Amyloidosis and Myeloma Unit, Hospital Clínic de Barcelona, Villarroel 170, 08036, Barcelona, Spain; [b] Institut D'Investigacions Biomèdiques August Pi I Sunyer, University of Barcelona, Spain
* Corresponding authors.
** Corresponding authors.
E-mail addresses: dfmoreno@clinic.cat (D.F.M.); cfernan1@clinic.cat (C.F.L.)

Hematol Oncol Clin N Am 37 (2023) 659–670
https://doi.org/10.1016/j.hoc.2023.04.002
0889-8588/23/© 2023 Elsevier Inc. All rights reserved.
hemonc.theclinics.com

techniques and highly sensitive polymerase chain reaction (PCR) assays, there is now an increasing number of options available to assess the genotypes of patients with WM. The availability of new methods to detect somatic mutations in WM has also made it possible to characterize and diagnose the disease, draw correlations with treatment responses, design new clinical trials, and redefine the prognostic risk in both asymptomatic and symptomatic patients.

Here, we review the current knowledge on the genomic landscape of WM and the clinical implications regarding diagnosis, treatment, and prognosis. We focus on recent advances using targeted or whole genome sequencing (WGS), novel PCR methods such as droplet digital PCR (ddPCR), the use of new potential sample sources like cell-free DNA (cfDNA), and the importance of defining the genotype to improve and personalize treatment.

Advances in the Biology of Waldenström Macroglobulinemia

The clinical need to analyze the genome of samples from patients with WM has been increasing during the last few years. Taking advantage of the wide availability of sequencing methods, we can now describe the mutation profile using bone marrow, peripheral blood, or even cfDNA samples. Moreover, recent novel approaches to assess the genome, such as single-cell sequencing, have brought us a wider picture of the clonal heterogeneity of this disease.

In this sense, there have been novel advances regarding the biology of WM. For example, detecting *MYD88* L265P early in B cell development gave more insight into the origin of the malignant clone. Cellular indexing of transcriptome and epitopes followed by sequencing has revealed that pre-B cells from WM had transcriptionally enriched pathways such as IL6-STAT3, similarly found in B cells. Furthermore, exome sequencing identified the *MYD88* L265P mutation in pre-B progenitors in the bone marrow of patients with WM and IgM MGUS.[7] Another study using single-cell DNA sequencing showed that *MYD88* L265P has been found not only in tumor B cells but also in B cell precursors and normal B lymphocytes from WM samples. Although *MYD88* L265P was detected early in B-cell development, the sole presence of the mutation could not drive lymphomagenesis in a mice model.[8] Altogether, these data demonstrated that small clonal alterations might originate during lymphopoiesis in WM. Still, the acquisition of *CXCR4* mutations, copy number alterations (CNAs), and del(6q) would confer a greater risk of clonal expansion, with the development of a phenotypically overt WM. This evolutionary model has also been proposed using a large targeted sequencing panel, by which CNAs were increasingly found in relapsed WM compared with stable WM. Leveraging WGS data, the same study identified gains in chromosome 12 early in the *MYD88*wt WM development, whereas other chromosomal gains occurred later.[9] These findings were similar to those reported in chronic lymphocytic leukemia and can serve as a basis for discovering potential biomarkers in a subset of patients with WM.

More recently, whole exome sequencing (WES) identified Spi-1 proto-oncogene (*SPI1*) Q226 E mutation in 6% of patients with WM. These results were later confirmed by either targeted or RNA sequencing on sorted tumor cells. *SPI1* encodes a transcription factor that activates gene expression in B-cell and myeloid-cell development. The mutant transcription factor binds to other promoter regions, which results in increased B-cell proliferation. *SPI1* Q226E mutation was associated with worse overall survival (OS) than the wild-type *SPI1* counterpart. Moreover, the study also reported a preclinical potential activity of BET (bromodomain and extraterminal) inhibitors or lenalidomide in *SPI1* Q226E WM, as MYC and IRF4-enriched signatures were associated with the mutant cases.[10]

Regarding the epigenome, the emerging methods to analyze it have also been applied in WM, giving more insights into the biology of the disease. By leveraging both a DNA methylation array and RNA sequencing in WM samples, a study could classify patients in 2 different subgroups, memory B-cell and plasma-cell-like showing different features. For instance, the memory B-cell-like group showed more *CXCR4* mutations and del(13q), whereas the plasma-cell-like group harbored more del(6q).[11]

The fact that highly prevalent somatic mutations in WM are also observed in early asymptomatic stages and the reported predisposition in family clusters make WM a model to study cancer biology and establish potential causal factors. In that context, genome-wide association studies can help understand the relationship between genetic variants and predisposition to cancer. In the case of WM, 2 loci (6p25.3 and 14q32.13) were associated with an increased risk of WM in a familial cluster of cases, later confirmed in a nonfamilial set. Both loci were closely related to previously known genes dysregulated in other lymphoid neoplasms, making them potential susceptibility regions.[12] Functional studies are needed to analyze the biological impact of these findings further.

After all these technological advances, the application of high-throughput technologies in WM has enabled to further disentangle the biology of the disease and to identify new biomarkers of disease progression with potential use in future clinical trials.

Impact on Clinical Phenotypes

From a clinical perspective, *MYD88* and *CXCR4* mutations can describe phenotypical characteristics in patients with WM. For instance, more than 60% of patients with WM harbor *MYD88*mut *CXCR4*wt genotype, associated with a moderate bone marrow lymphoplasmacytic infiltrate and high serum IgM level. *MYD88*mut *CXCR4*mut is the second most common genotype (approximately 30%–40% of patients with WM). It has been associated with higher bone marrow involvement and serum IgM level, thus observing a higher incidence of hyperviscosity.[3] Different gene-expression profiling methods confirmed that a *CXCR4* signature was associated with this clinical phenotype.[13,14]

Among the *CXCR4* S338* mutations reported in WM, C>G transversion is the most frequently reported. This mutation has been associated with both bone marrow homing of lymphoplasmacytic cells and extramedullary dissemination, explaining in part the clinical phenotype of *CXCR4*mut patients.[15]

As previously mentioned, the epigenetic characterization of WM into a memory B-cell and plasma-cell-like groups also revealed differential clinical characteristics. Memory B-cell-like WM cases were associated with increased thrombocytopenia and splenomegaly. These patients also exhibited a higher variant allele frequency of *CXCR4* mutations. However, plasma-cell-like cases showed differences in the morphology of tumor cells and CNAs but no clinical phenotype was distinctive.[11]

Finally, less than 10% of patients with WM are *MYD88*wt *CXCR4*wt. This genotype is associated with an increased prevalence of lymphadenopathy and a higher risk for transformation to a diffuse large B-cell lymphoma (DLBCL).[16] Using WES, *MYD88*wt cases harbored mutations that are known to trigger NF-Kb activation or are involved in epigenomic dysregulation and DNA damage repair. For instance, mutations in *TBL1XR1* were identified in *MYD88*wt WM cases, also reported in other B-cell lymphomas with aggressive presentation.[17] Yet caution is needed in *MYD88*wt WM cases, as a proportion of them might still show a different diagnosis, which includes IgM-secreting marginal zone lymphoma or IgM multiple myeloma.[16]

Treatment Response According to the Mutation Status

Given that there are associations between the genotypes and the clinical presentation of patients with WM, efforts have been made to include the mutation status in the design of clinical trials. Although there are no meta-analyses to disentangle the impact of genotypes on treatment effect, the general overview is that *MYD88*wt patients achieved lower overall response rate (ORR), followed by those with concomitant *MYD88* and *CXCR4* mutations. A plausible explanation is that *MYD88*wt WM cases showed a mutation profile similar to some aggressive B-cell lymphomas.[17] However, *CXCR4* mutations confer a higher disease burden in the *MYD88*mut cases.[15]

In fact, it has been reported that ORR to ibrutinib was higher in *MYD88*mut patients with or without concomitant *CXCR4* mutations compared with *MYD88*wt.[18] Moreover, *MYD88*wt cases achieved lower ORR than the other 2 genotypes in the study that combined ibrutinib with rituximab.[19] When using second-generation Bruton tyrosine kinase (BTK) inhibitors, acalabrutinib also showed higher ORR in *MYD88*mut patients compared with wild type.[20] Retrospective studies analyzing the role of *CXCR4* mutations on ibrutinib response have also reported that nonsense *CXCR4*mut patients achieved lower major response rates compared with frameshift *CXCR4*mut.[21] These results again favored the importance of testing for *CXCR4* S338* mutations because the nonsense mutations might associate with a less functional protein. Moreover, the mutation burden of *CXCR4* S338* has been also associated with reduced very good partial response rates in patients who received ibrutinib monotherapy.[21] The lower responses in *MYD88*mut *CXCR4*mut showed in the trials using ibrutinib monotherapy could be partially improved by incorporating rituximab.[19]

Similarly, patients treated with zanubrutinib achieved a higher partial response or better rates in *MYD88*mut *CXCR4*wt and *MYD88*mut *CXCR4*mut patients compared with wild type.[22] Venetoclax, a B-cell lymphoma 2 (BCL2) inhibitor, had a similar trend to better ORR in *MYD88*mut *CXCR4*wt patients compared with those harboring *CXCR4* mutations.[23] Among other new agents, the combination of ixazomib, dexamethasone, and rituximab reported higher ORR in *MYD88*mut *CXCR4*wt and *MYD88*mut *CXCR4*mut, with a slightly inferior proportion of response in the patients of the latter group.[24]

As we previously exposed, *CXCR4* mutations might confer not only a greater disease burden but also a trend to lower response rates. To mitigate this problem, new agents against *CXCR4* (ulocuplumab or mavorixafor) have shown promising results in *MYD88*mut *CXCR4*mut patients.[25,26] Noncovalent BTK inhibitors (pirtobrutinib) and the combination of acalabrutinib or venetoclax with rituximab are being evaluated in clinical trials in patients with WM, thus giving further insights into the impact of genotypes on treatment effects.

Prognosis According to Genotypes in Waldenström Macroglobulinemia

Classification of patients with WM according to genotype has been able to draw associations with OS. An early analysis doing both AS-PCR and Sanger sequencing for *MYD88* L265P and *CXCR4* mutations in bone marrow samples from 174 patients with WM showed that OS was shorter in *MYD88*wt patients compared with those harboring the L265P mutation.[3] Moreover, the updated analysis after a longer median follow-up confirmed these results. Thus, the 10-year estimated OS for *MYD88*wt and *MYD88*mut patients was 73% and 90%, respectively.[16] In both studies, the co-occurrence of *CXCR4* mutations in *MYD88*mut patients did not affect OS. As explained above, *MYD88*wt patients share a certain mutation profile with other aggressive B-cell lymphomas.[17] These findings were also translated into a higher incidence of transformation to DLBCL with an ominous prognosis.[16]

Regarding progression-free survival (PFS), *MYD88*wt patients had shorter PFS followed by *MYD88*mut *CXCR4*mut patients treated with ibrutinib monotherapy.[18,27] Similar PFS was observed in the case of ibrutinib with rituximab regardless of mutation status.[19] Patients treated with venetoclax and ixazomib, dexamethasone and rituximab reported *MYD88* mutations in all patients, and the co-occurrence of *CXCR4* mutations did not affect PFS in both studies.[24] Similarly, the combination of obinutuzumab and idelalisib showed no differences in PFS regarding the *CXCR4* mutation status; however, 24% of the whole series harbored *TP53* mutations, and they had a trend to worse impact.[28]

However, the availability of genotyping early asymptomatic stages has increased in the last years, further elucidating the risk of progression to symptomatic disease. The interest remains in the fact that *MYD88* and/or *CXCR4* mutations can model the progression in IgM MGUS and SWM. In this scenario, *MYD88* L265P was found in 54% of a series of patients with IgM MGUS assessed by AS-PCR showing a shorter PFS after a median follow-up of 83 months.[29] Similarly, other study using ddPCR reported 64% and 35% of *MYD88* L265P and *CXCR4* S338* mutations prevalence in patients with IgM MGUS, showing an increased incidence of progression to symptomatic disease in those cases with high allele burden.[30] In the case of SWM, 2 studies using AS-PCR showed that *MYD88*wt patients had shorter PFS than *MYD88*mut.[31,32] More recently, it was reported that the co-occurrence of *MYD88* L265P and *CXCR4* S338* mutations and a high allele burden increased the probability of progression in SWM leveraging ddPCR technology.[30]

Another biomarker that negatively affects outcomes in patients with WM is del(6q). A study reported a prevalence of 4%, 9%, and 30% of del(6q) in IgM MGUS, SWM, and symptomatic patients with WM, respectively. Patients harboring del(6q) had a shorter time to disease progression in the asymptomatic stages. Meanwhile, symptomatic patients with WM with del(6q) had a shorter time to next treatment. Irrespective of diagnosis, OS was shorter in all groups with del(6q).[33]

Thus, the absence of mutations in *MYD88* confers a higher risk of transformation to an aggressive B-cell lymphoma to patients with WM and is associated with a shorter OS compared with the other 2 genotypes. *CXCR4*mut status apparently affects treatment response, especially after BTK inhibitors but with no clear impact on OS. In case of the asymptomatic stages, as most samples have a relatively lower disease burden, there is a great dependency on the technology used to analyze somatic mutations. It seems that higher tumor burden could be associated with shorter time to symptomatic disease.

New Technologies to Assess the Genotypes of Waldenström Macroglobulinemia

Since the detection of *MYD88* L265P in WM using WGS in selected CD19+ bone marrow cells,[2] designing PCR-based methods has helped expand and reproduce the mutation detection among different centers around the world. **Fig. 1** summarizes the most common sample sources used to analyze mutations or other genomic alterations in WM. Using CD19+ selected samples, unselected bone marrow, or even peripheral blood samples, AS-PCR has proven to achieve high sensitivity and specificity to detect *MYD88* L265P.[4] In the case of *CXCR4*, the attention has been focused on the nonsense S338* c.1013 C > G and c.1013 C > A mutations. AS-PCR assays to test both mutations have also been developed and reproduced; however, as most of them are subclonal, sorting CD19+ bone marrow cells was an important step before PCR amplification.[5] More recently, sequencing targeted genes using different platforms has enabled to assess other mutations already described before by WGS or WES. This technology partially compensates for cost issues to sequence a genome,

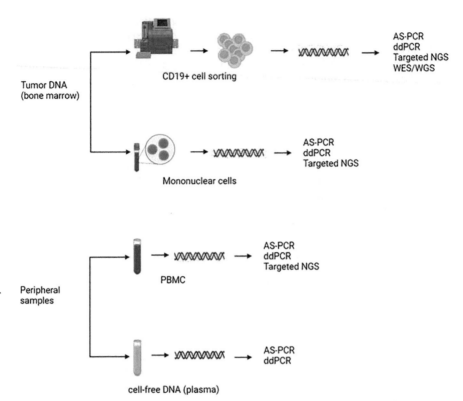

Fig. 1. Samples commonly used for the analysis of genomic alterations of patients with WM. Direct tumor DNA can be obtained from bone marrow samples, followed by CD19+ sorting or enrichment and DNA extraction. Another approach is to use bone marrow mononuclear cells (figure above). Peripheral samples can be processed to obtain peripheral blood mononuclear cells (PBMC) followed by DNA extraction, or plasma samples can be processed to obtain cfDNA (figure below). AS-PCR, allele-specific polymerase chain reaction; ddPCR, droplet digital polymerase chain reaction; NGS, next-generation sequencing; WES, whole exome sequencing; WGS, whole genome sequencing.

achieving high sensitivity. However, very small subclones are difficult to detect. In this sense, customizable features before sequencing can achieve deeper resolution, thus increasing the costs.[34] **Table 1** summarizes studies where AS-PCR was used in IgM MGUS and WM to detect *MYD88* L265P and *CXCR4* S338* mutations. As observed, there is a wide variation of mutation-detection rates when using unselected or selected CD19+ bone marrow or peripheral blood samples in IgM MGUS.

Recently, based partially on the somehow patchy bone marrow infiltration and the need to detect mutations bypassing a bone marrow biopsy, cfDNA is becoming an important source under investigation. Although not yet standardized internationally, several studies have reported the detection of both *MYD88* L265P and *CXCR4* S338* mutations with AS-PCR. **Table 2** also summarizes studies that used cfDNA as a source of material.

More lately, and because of the need to achieve an even deeper resolution to detect somatic mutations, some groups have focused on ddPCR. This technology has already achieved higher sensitivity than AS-PCR, thus replacing the prior CD19+ sorting step. This step is particularly problematic in 3 situations: very small clones in IgM

Table 1
Summary of studies using bone marrow samples as a source of material for testing *MYD88* and *CXCR4* mutations

Studies Using Bone Marrow Samples	MYD88mut		CXCR4mut	
	IgM MGUS	WM	IgM MGUS	WM
Treon et al,[2] 2012 Sanger on CD19+ cells	2/21 (10%)	49/54 (91%)	-	-
Xu et al,[4] 2013 AS-PCR on CD19+ cells	13/24 (54%)	97/104 (93%)	-	-
Jiménez et al,[38] 2013 ASO-PCR on unsorted cells	27/31 (87%)	101/117 (86%)	-	-
Treon et al,[3] 2014 AS-PCR on CD19+ cells for MYD88 Sanger on CD19+ cells for CXCR4	-	158/175 (90%)	-	51/175 (29%)
Varettoni et al,[39] 2013 AS-PCR on unsorted cells	36/77 (47%)	58/58 (100%)	-	-
Xu et al,[40] 2015 AS-PCR on CD19+ cells Sanger on CD19+ cells	6/12 (50%)	97/102 (95%)	2/12 (17%)	44/102 (43%)
Varettoni et al,[41] 2017 AS-PCR on CD19+ cells for MYD88 Sanger on CD19+ cells for CXCR4	78/130 (60%)	112/130 (86%)	5/130 (4%)	29/130 (22%)
Drandi et al,[42] 2018 ddPCR on unsorted cells	-	109/112 (97%)	-	-
Ferrante et al,[35] 2021 ddPCR on unsorted cells	54/62 (87%)	93/97 (96%)	-	-
Moreno et al,[30] 2022[a] ddPCR on unsorted cells	54/84 (64%)	45/55 (82%)	21/54 (39%)	21/42 (50%)

The percentage is the mutation detection prevalence reported.
Abbreviations: AS-PCR, allele-specific polymerase chain reaction; ASO-PCR, allele-specific oligonucleotide polymerase chain reaction; ddPCR, droplet digital polymerase chain reaction; MGUS, monoclonal gammopathy of undetermined significance; SWM, smoldering Waldenström macroglobulinemia; WM, Waldenström macroglobulinemia.
[a] These data refer only to smoldering Waldenström macroglobulinemia patients.

Table 2
Summary of studies using cell-free DNA as source of material for testing *MYD88* and *CXCR4* mutations

Studies Using Cell-free DNA Samples	MYD88^mut		CXCR4^mut	
	IgM MGUS	WM	IgM MGUS	WM
Drandi et al,[42] 2018 ddPCR	-	53/60 (88%)	-	-
Wu et al,[43] 2020 AS-PCR	-	23/27 (85%)	-	1/27 (4%)
Demos et al,[44] 2021 AS-PCR	-	20/28 (71%)	-	4/23 (17%)
Ferrante et al,[35] 2021 ddPCR	3/4 (75%)	25/32 (78%)	-	-
Moreno et al,[30] 2022[a] ddPCR	8/21 (38%)	10/16 (63%)	0	1/10 (10%)

The percentage is the mutation detection prevalence reported.

Abbreviations: AS-PCR, allele specific polymerase chain reaction; ddPCR, droplet digital polymerase chain reaction; MGUS, monoclonal gammopathy of undetermined significance; SWM, smoldering Waldenström macroglobulinemia; WM, Waldenström macroglobulinemia.

[a] These data refer only to smoldering Waldenström macroglobulinemia patients.

MGUS or minimal residual disease assessment in WM, subclonality of *CXCR4* mutations, and using cfDNA as samples. Because ddPCR can achieve absolute quantification of a mutation, it has shown promising results as a mutation detection method and a biomarker of disease progression in its early stages. For instance, a study reported that *MYD88* L265P mutation was detected in more cases in IgM MGUS (up to 64%) using ddPCR compared with AS-PCR in unsorted bone marrow samples.[30] Moreover, a comparative study that analyzed sorted CD19+ versus unsorted samples described no differences in detecting the *MYD88* L265P mutation using ddPCR.[35] Regarding *CXCR4* mutations, ddPCR detected S338* mutations in up to 35% of patients with IgM MGUS without prior CD19+ sorting step.[30] Previously, others reported *CXCR4* mutations in 17%[5] and 29%[36] of CD19+ sorted IgM MGUS samples using AS-PCR and/or Sanger sequencing.

Another recent PCR-based method reported is competitive allele-specific PCR (Cast-PCR). Cast-PCR can work with very low amounts of DNA either on tumoral or cfDNA samples and can properly quantify the mutation burden. Although the limit of detection of Cast-PCR to detect *MYD88* L265P was 0.1%, between the canonical AS-PCR (1%) and ddPCR (0.05%), the ability to work with low amounts of DNA made it a potential candidate to assess cfDNA samples.[37]

As we rely on the continuous advances of high-throughput technologies to detect somatic mutations in cancer, promising tools are guaranteed regarding deeper sensitivity for *MYD88* L265P and *CXCR4* S338* mutations. The increasing availability of new methods also necessitates standardizing mutation detection in WM. Further studies will confirm the reproducibility of the results for *CXCR4* mutations using ddPCR in WM.

SUMMARY

Genotype testing is an important step to a better diagnosis of patients with WM, for predicting disease progression in IgM MGUS or SWM, evaluating treatment response, and designing clinical trials. The genotypes based on *MYD88* and *CXCR4* mutations are translated into clinical characteristics and can affect the PFS and OS of patients with WM. Advances to increase depth of mutation detection is critical, as well as a need to standardize methods among different centers. ddPCR has proven to be a reliable technique to analyze *MYD88* and *CXCR4* mutations in WM using either bone marrow or cfDNA samples and can obviate the CD19+ sorting step.

CLINICS CARE POINTS

- *MYD88* and *CXCR4* mutations are critical in the biology of WM. *MYD88* L265P is an early event during the evolution of the lymphoplasmacytic clone. *CXCR4* S338* mutations are subclonal to MYD88 and confer greater risk of disease progression.

- More than 90% and up to 40% of patients with WM harbor *MYD88* and *CXCR4* mutations, respectively. Caution should be taken in *MYD88*wt patients because some of them might have an alternative diagnosis or are in greater risk of transformation to aggressive lymphomas.

- Novel techniques can achieve higher sensitivity to detect somatic mutations, along with precise quantification of the mutation burden. AS-PCR have demonstrated reproducible results among different studies, whereas ddPCR is an emerging technology that can overtake detection issues in samples with very-low tumor burden (ie, IgM MGUS, minimal residual disease follow-up, use of cfDNA, among others).

- *MYD88* and *CXCR4* mutations translate into a clinical phenotype in patients with WM. *CXCR4*mut patients show more serum IgM, increased prevalence of hyperviscosity, and higher bone marrow infiltration.

- Genotype testing is crucial in the inclusion for clinical trials and may also contribute to evaluate treatment response. *MYD88*mut patients show higher ORRs to BTK inhibitors compared with *MYD88*wt, with a longer median OS.

DISCLOSURES

D.F. Moreno: Travel grants and honoraria by Janssen. C. Fernández de Larrea: Advisory boards from Amgen, Janssen, and BMS; research grants from Janssen, BMS, Takeda, and Amgen; honoraria for lectures: BMS, Takeda, Sanofi, Amgen, Janssen, GSK, and Beigene.

REFERENCES

1. Hunter ZR, Xu L, Yang G, et al. The genomic landscape of Waldenstrom macroglobulinemia is characterized by highly recurring MYD88 and WHIM-like CXCR4 mutations, and small somatic deletions associated with B-cell lymphomagenesis. Blood 2014;123(11):1637–46.
2. Treon SP, Xu L, Yang G, et al. MYD88 L265P Somatic Mutation in Waldenström's Macroglobulinemia. N Engl J Med 2012;367(9):826–33.
3. Treon SP, Cao Y, Xu L, et al. Somatic mutations in MYD88 and CXCR4 are determinants of clinical presentation and overall survival in Waldenstrom macroglobulinemia. Blood 2014;123(18):2791–6.
4. Xu L, Hunter ZR, Yang G, et al. MYD88 L265P in Waldenstrom macroglobulinemia, immunoglobulin M monoclonal gammopathy, and other B-cell lymphoproliferative disorders using conventional and quantitative allele-specific polymerase chain reaction. Blood 2013;121(11):2051–8.
5. Xu L, Hunter ZR, Tsakmaklis N, et al. Clonal architecture of CXCR4 WHIM-like mutations in Waldenström Macroglobulinaemia. Br J Haematol 2016;172(5):735–44.

6. Treon SP, Xu L, Guerrera ML, et al. Genomic Landscape of Waldenström Macroglobulinemia and Its Impact on Treatment Strategies. J Clin Orthod 2020;38(11): 1198–208.

7. Kaushal A, Nooka AK, Carr AR, et al. Aberrant Extrafollicular B Cells, Immune Dysfunction, Myeloid Inflammation, and MyD88-Mutant Progenitors Precede Waldenstrom Macroglobulinemia. Blood Cancer Discov 2021 Nov;2(6):600–15.

8. Rodriguez S, Celay J, Goicoechea I, et al. Preneoplastic somatic mutations including MYD88 L265P in lymphoplasmacytic lymphoma. Sci Adv 2022;8(3): eabl4644.

9. Maclachlan KH, Bagratuni T, Kastritis E, et al. Waldenström Macroglobulinemia Whole Genome Reveals Prolonged Germinal Center Activity and Late Copy Number Aberrations. Blood Advances 2022;7(6):971–81.

10. Roos-Weil D, Decaudin C, Armand M, et al. A Recurrent Activating Missense Mutation in Waldenström Macroglobulinemia Affects the DNA Binding of the ETS Transcription Factor SPI1 and Enhances Proliferation. Cancer Discov 2019;9(6): 796–811.

11. Roos-Weil D, Giacopelli B, Armand M, et al. Identification of two DNA methylation subtypes of Waldenström's macroglobulinemia with plasma and memory B cell features. Blood 2020;136(5):585–95.

12. McMaster ML, Berndt SI, Zhang J, et al. Two high-risk susceptibility loci at 6p25.3 and 14q32.13 for Waldenström macroglobulinemia. Nat Commun 2018;9(1): 4182.

13. Hunter ZR, Xu L, Yang G, et al. Transcriptome sequencing reveals a profile that corresponds to genomic variants in Waldenström macroglobulinemia. Blood 2016;128(6):827–38.

14. Poulain S, Roumier C, Venet-Caillault A, et al. Genomic Landscape of CXCR4 Mutations in Waldenström Macroglobulinemia. Clin Cancer Res 2016;22(6):1480–8.

15. Roccaro AM, Sacco A, Jimenez C, et al. C1013G/CXCR4 acts as a driver mutation of tumor progression and modulator of drug resistance in lymphoplasmacytic lymphoma. Blood 2014;123(26):4120–31.

16. Treon SP, Gustine J, Xu L, et al. MYD88 wild-type Waldenstrom Macroglobulinaemia: differential diagnosis, risk of histological transformation, and overall survival. Br J Haematol 2018;180(3):374–80.

17. Hunter ZR, Xu L, Tsakmaklis N, et al. Insights into the genomic landscape of MYD88 wild-type Waldenström macroglobulinemia. Blood Advances 2018; 2(21):2937–46.

18. Treon SP, Tripsas CK, Meid K, et al. Ibrutinib in Previously Treated Waldenström's Macroglobulinemia. N Engl J Med 2015;372(15):1430–40.

19. Buske C, Tedeschi A, Trotman J, et al. Ibrutinib Plus Rituximab Versus Placebo Plus Rituximab for Waldenström's Macroglobulinemia: Final Analysis From the Randomized Phase III iNNOVATE Study. J Clin Orthod 2022;40(1):52–62.

20. Owen RG, McCarthy H, Rule S, et al. Acalabrutinib monotherapy in patients with Waldenström macroglobulinemia: a single-arm, multicentre, phase 2 study. Lancet Haematology 2020;7(2):e112–21.

21. Castillo JJ, Xu L, Gustine JN, et al. CXCR4 mutation subtypes impact response and survival outcomes in patients with Waldenström macroglobulinaemia treated with ibrutinib. Br J Haematol 2019;187(3):356–63.

22. Tam CS, Opat S, D'Sa S, et al. A randomized phase 3 trial of zanubrutinib vs ibrutinib in symptomatic Waldenström macroglobulinemia: the ASPEN study. Blood 2020;136(18):2038–50.

23. Castillo JJ, Allan JN, Siddiqi T, et al. Venetoclax in Previously Treated Waldenström Macroglobulinemia. J Clin Orthod 2022;40(1):63–71.
24. Castillo JJ, Meid K, Flynn CA, et al. Ixazomib, dexamethasone, and rituximab in treatment-naive patients with Waldenström macroglobulinemia: long-term follow-up. Blood Advances 2020;4(16):3952–9.
25. Treon SP, Meid K, Hunter ZR, et al. Phase 1 study of ibrutinib and the CXCR4 antagonist ulocuplumab in CXCR4-mutated Waldenström macroglobulinemia. Blood 2021;138(17):1535–9.
26. Treon SP, Buske C, Thomas SK, et al. Preliminary Clinical Response Data from a Phase 1b Study of Mavorixafor in Combination with Ibrutinib in Patients with Waldenström's Macroglobulinemia with *MYD88* and *CXCR4* Mutations. Blood 2021; 138(Supplement 1):1362.
27. Treon SP, Meid K, Gustine J, et al. Long-Term Follow-Up of Ibrutinib Monotherapy in Symptomatic, Previously Treated Patients With Waldenström Macroglobulinemia. J Clin Orthod 2021;39(6):565–75.
28. Tomowiak C, Poulain S, Herbaux C, et al. Obinutuzumab and idelalisib in symptomatic patients with relapsed/refractory Waldenström macroglobulinemia. Blood Advances 2021;5(9):2438–46.
29. Varettoni M, Zibellini S, Boveri E, et al. A risk-stratification model based on the initial concentration of the serum monoclonal protein and *MYD 88* mutation status identifies a subset of patients with IgM monoclonal gammopathy of undetermined significance at high risk of progression to Waldenström macroglobulinaemia or other lymphoproliferative disorders. Br J Haematol 2019;187(4):441–6.
30. Moreno DF, López-Guerra M, Paz S, et al. Prognostic impact of MYD88 and CXCR4 mutations assessed by droplet digital polymerase chain reaction in IgM monoclonal gammopathy of undetermined significance and smouldering Waldenström macroglobulinaemia. Br J Haematol 2022;bjh:18502.
31. Bustoros M, Sklavenitis-Pistofidis R, Kapoor P, et al. Progression Risk Stratification of Asymptomatic Waldenström Macroglobulinemia. J Clin Oncol 2019;19: 00394.
32. Zanwar S, Abeykoon JP, Ansell SM, et al. Disease outcomes and biomarkers of progression in smouldering Waldenström macroglobulinaemia. Br J Haematol 2021;195(2):210–6.
33. García-Sanz R, Dogliotti I, Zaccaria GM, et al. 6q deletion in Waldenström macroglobulinaemia negatively affects time to transformation and survival. Br J Haematol 2021;192(5):843–52.
34. Berger MF, Mardis ER. The emerging clinical relevance of genomics in cancer medicine. Nat Rev Clin Oncol 2018;15(6):353–65.
35. Ferrante M, Furlan D, Zibellini S, et al. MYD88L265P Detection in IgM Monoclonal Gammopathies: Methodological Considerations for Routine Implementation. Diagnostics 2021;11(5):779.
36. Bagratuni T, Ntanasis-Stathopoulos I, Gavriatopoulou M, et al. Detection of MYD88 and CXCR4 mutations in cell-free DNA of patients with IgM monoclonal gammopathies. Leukemia 2018;32(12):2617–25.
37. Bagratuni T, Markou A, Patseas D, et al. Determination of MYD88[L265P] mutation fraction in IgM monoclonal gammopathies. Blood Advances 2022;6(1):189–99.
38. Jiménez C, Sebastián E, Chillón MC, et al. MYD88 L265P is a marker highly characteristic of, but not restricted to, Waldenström's macroglobulinemia. Leukemia 2013;27(8):1722–8.

39. Varettoni M, Arcaini L, Zibellini S, et al. Prevalence and clinical significance of the MYD88 (L265P) somatic mutation in Waldenstrom's macroglobulinemia and related lymphoid neoplasms. Blood 2013;121(13):2522–8.

40. Xu L, Hunter ZR, Tsakmaklis N, et al. Clonal architecture of CXCR4 WHIM-like mutations in Waldenström Macroglobulinaemia. Br J Haematol 2016;172(5):735–44.

41. Varettoni M, Zibellini S, Defrancesco I, et al. Pattern of somatic mutations in patients with Waldenström macroglobulinemia or IgM monoclonal gammopathy of undetermined significance. Haematologica 2017;102(12):2077–85.

42. Drandi D, Genuardi E, Dogliotti I, et al. Highly sensitive MYD88L265P mutation detection by droplet digital polymerase chain reaction in Waldenström macroglobulinemia. Haematologica 2018;103(6):1029–37.

43. Wu YY, Jia MN, Cai H, et al. Detection of the MYD88L265P and CXCR4S338X mutations by cell-free DNA in Waldenström macroglobulinemia. Ann Hematol 2020; 99(8):1763–9.

44. Demos MG, Hunter ZR, Xu L, et al. Cell-free DNA analysis for detection of MYD88L265P and CXCR4S338X mutations in Waldenström macroglobulinemia. Am J Hematol 2021;96(7):E250–3.

Frontline Management of Waldenström Macroglobulinemia with Chemoimmunotherapy

Prashant Kapoor, MD*, Jonas Paludo, MD,
Jithma P. Abeykoon, MD**

KEYWORDS

- IgM lymphoplasmacytic lymphoma • Alkylating agents • Purine analogs
- Monoclonal antibodies • Limited-duration treatment

KEY POINTS

- Chemoimmunotherapy is a valuable and effective frontline approach for the management of patients with Waldenström macroglobulinemia.
- Alkylator-based chemotherapy with rituximab, especially bendamustine and rituximab doublet is highly active and commonly used in the treatment of Waldenstrom macroglobulinemia.
- The outcome of patients with Waldenström macroglobulinemia receiving chemoimmunotherapy is independent of their MYD88 mutation status.
- The finite duration of chemoimmunotherapy is particularly appealing to patients, given that the majority of toxicities resolve with completion of treatment.

INTRODUCTION

Waldenström Macroglobulinemia (WM) is a B-cell, IgM-secreting lymphoplasmacytic lymphoma (LPL), with an incidence of 1500–2000 new cases per year in the United States.[1–3] The median age at presentation is approximately 70 years and the disease is predominantly encountered among Caucasians. Despite remarkable advances in the field, WM remains incurable, with no benefit of early therapeutic intervention among the asymptomatic, incidentally diagnosed patients, without indications to treat. Moreover, patients with smoldering WM, managed with active surveillance alone, show comparable survival to the age- and sex-matched general population.[4] Therefore, in the absence of data supporting the benefit of early use of WM-directed therapy,

Division of Hematology, Mayo Clinic, 200 First Street Southwest, Rochester, MN 55905, USA
* Corresponding author.
** Corresponding author.
E-mail addresses: kapoor.prashant@mayo.edu (P.K.); abeykoon.jithma@mayo.edu (J.P.A.)

Hematol Oncol Clin N Am 37 (2023) 671–687
https://doi.org/10.1016/j.hoc.2023.04.003
0889-8588/23/© 2023 Elsevier Inc. All rights reserved.

intervention is best reserved for patients with active disease exhibiting unrelenting symptoms or significant cytopenias attributable to underlying WM. As curative therapies are lacking, palliation of symptoms, with disease control, and preservation of the quality of life have become overarching goals of the management of WM. When the patients with WM meet the indications for treatment, outside of clinical trials, they are typically offered one of the 3 approaches (i) fixed-duration chemoimmunotherapy (CIT), (ii) fixed-duration proteasome-inhibitor (PI)-based approach, or (iii) Bruton tyrosine kinase (BTK)-inhibitor-based treatment given continuously until progression or intolerable treatment-emergent toxicity. This review focuses on the CIT-based approaches for patients with previously untreated WM.

The preponderance of evidence in WM that has shaped our current approach was gathered either from subset analyses exclusively focused on WM patients within the larger randomized controlled trials of indolent lymphomas, or single-arm phase 2 trials and retrospective studies focussing on patients with WM. For a long time, limited-duration chemotherapy has been the linchpin of managing symptomatic WM. With the recognition of the merits of integrating anti-CD20 monoclonal antibodies into the existing chemotherapy backbones, CIT became a widely adopted strategy. Over time, as evidence from the use of CIT accumulated (**Fig. 1**), clinicians became more adept at managing this rare non-Hodgkin lymphoma. Fixed-duration anti-CD20 plus PI-based combinations have also been developed, but did not supplant CIT, probably due to the high rates of PI-associated neurotoxicity, particularly with bortezomib, among patients with WM. More recently, continuous BTKi-based therapies have offered an alternative approach to CIT although randomized trials comparing the 2 vastly different strategies remain absent.

Rituximab is a chimeric anti-CD20 monoclonal antibody with substantial clinical activity in WM, a malignancy with variable CD20 expression. Single-agent response

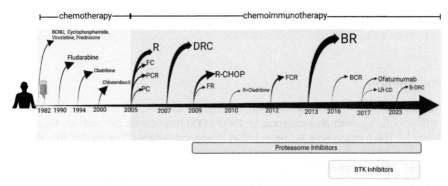

Fig. 1. Evolution of Chemoimmunotherapy in Waldenström Macroglobulinemia. The font sizes and the arrow width depict the impact of the respective regimens in the frontline setting. The time points on the horizontal axis represent the year of the publication of the initial clinical trial(s) with the specific regimens. The horizontal bars at the bottom show the time interval during which other classes of frequently used agents were developed and continue to be used in WM. Created with BioRender.com. BCNU, carmustine; BCR, bortezomib, cyclophosphamide, and dexamethasone; B-DRC, bortezomib, dexamethasone, rituximab, and cyclophosphamide; BR, bendamustine, and rituximab; BTK, Bruton's tyrosine kinase; DRC, dexamethasone, rituximab, and cyclophosphamide; FC, fludarabine, and cyclophosphamide; FCR, fludarabine, cyclophosphamide, and rituximab; FR, fludarabine and rituximab; LR-CD, lenalidomide, rituximab, cyclophosphamide, and dexamethasone; PC, pentostatin, and cyclophosphamide; PCR, pentostatin, cyclophosphamide, and rituximab; R, rituximab; R-CHOP, rituximab, cyclophosphamide, doxorubicin, vincristine, and prednisone.

rates of 30% to 50% have been observed in patients with treatment naïve WM.[5] Ofatumumab, another anti-CD20 monoclonal antibody, targets a different epitope of CD20 surface antigen and has more potent complement-dependent cytotoxicity than its predecessor, rituximab. As it is a fully human antibody, it is often used for patients who are rituximab intolerant, although scant prospective data support this approach. In a single-arm phase 2 trial, ofatumumab monotherapy has led to an overall response rate (ORR) of 67% among previously untreated WM (n = 9), with somewhat lower rates of IgM flare compared with rituximab.[6] In cross-trial comparisons, combination CIT regimens, for example, bendamustine or cyclophosphamide and anti-CD20 antibody, have shown superior disease control compared with anti-CD20 monotherapy, albeit at the cost of increased toxicity.

ALKYLATING AGENT-BASED REGIMENS

The German Low-Grade Lymphoma Study Group (GLSG) data published in 2009 underscored the value of concurrently using rituximab with conventional chemotherapy and put R-CHOP as one of the viable alternatives for the treatment of WM in medically fit patients.[7] The GLSG trial was an open-label, phase 3 study involving treatment naïve patients with advanced-stage indolent lymphomas (follicular lymphoma, LPL and mantle cell lymphoma). Buske and colleagues reported on the subset analysis of patients with active WM (n = 48 of 64 evaluable patients with LPL) who were randomly assigned in the GLSG study to receive CHOP (cyclophosphamide, doxorubicin, vincristine, and prednisone; n = 25) or rituximab plus CHOP (n = 23) for 4 to 8 3-week cycles. The median age of patients at study entry was 61 (range 37–78) years. Although the complete remission (CR) rates were disappointingly low and similar between the 2 regimens (9% vs 4%; P = .60), a considerably higher ORR was observed with R-CHOP (91%) compared with CHOP alone (60%; P = .019) which translated into a substantially longer time-to-treatment failure (TTF, the primary endpoint of the study) with R-CHOP (median 63 months) compared to with the CHOP arm (median 22 months, P = .024).[7] Alopecia, mucositis, infections, nausea, and vomiting comprised the main nonhematological toxicities, occurring at similar frequencies with both regimens, though the sample size was small to detect differences.[7]

A subsequent single-arm phase 2 Eastern Cooperative Oncology Group (ECOG) trial, E1A02, confirmed the high degree of ORR achieved with the R-CHOP regimen (100%), with a major response rate (MRR) of 91%, and at the short median follow-up of approximately 18 months. The median duration of response (DOR) was not reached.[8] This study was activated in 2004 after the GLSG trial had completed its accrual but was prematurely closed due to poor enrollment (n = 16), highlighting the need for international collaboration, with close involvement of advocacy groups for successfully bringing the trials involving a rare malignancy such as WM to fruition.

Patients with WM are inherently predisposed to peripheral neuropathy. Although there were no major differences encountered in the treatment-emergent toxicities between the 2 regimens in the GLSG substudy, myelosuppression, predominantly neutropenia, and vincristine-induced neurotoxicity (encountered in nearly 50% of the patients despite omission of the drug in the subsequent cycles at first signs of neuropathy) make the CHOP-based regimens unappealing, particularly for the frail or less medically fit patients with WM.[9] On the other hand, the dexamethasone, rituximab, and cyclophosphamide (DRC) regimen, first introduced by the Greek Group, retained the steroid (dexamethasone, instead of prednisone), CD20-directed therapy (rituximab) and the alkylator (cyclophosphamide given orally), but eliminated the vinca alkaloid (vincristine) and the anthracycline (doxorubicin), thereby making it more appealing than R-CHOP for the less-fit patient population. In a single-arm phase 2 trial, 72 patients with previously untreated WM were given the DRC regimen.[10,11] This study reported an ORR of 83%, with 67% of these patients achieving a partial response (PR) and 7% achieving a CR. The median progression-free survival (PFS) was 35 months (vs 23 months with rituximab single-agent), the median time-to-next treatment was 51 months and the median overall survival (OS) was 95 months (8-year OS rate of 47%).[10] Notably, approximately 3% of patients developed myelodysplastic syndrome (MDS) during a median follow-up period of 8 years (range 7–10 years), and ~10% transformed to diffuse large B-cell lymphoma (DLBCL). The regimen was well tolerated, particularly with low rates of neutropenia and thrombocytopenia. It has, however, not been prospectively compared with R-CHOP (no longer commonly used outside of histologic transformation to DLBCL) or BR.

Soon after the promising results of the DRC study were initially reported, the Mayo Clinic Group examined the incremental value of incorporating lenalidomide (20 mg PO, days 1–21) into the modified DRC backbone in a single-arm phase 2 trial for indolent lymphomas. Among the evaluable patients with WM, the ORR was 80%, (7% CR and 73% PR). The median PFS for the cohort of patients with WM was 38 months and the median OS had not been reached. While in this trial, lenalidomide could be safely combined with DRC, the results did not show an advantage of using it concurrently.[12] More recently, the results of ECWM-1 trial that again built upon the DRC backbone were published. The ECWM-1 (NCT01788020) study, a randomized-controlled phase 3 clinical trial involving patients with previously untreated WM, assessed the effect of adding bortezomib, a first-generation proteasome inhibitor with established activity in WM, to a modified DRC regimen, administered once every 4 weeks with subcutaneous rituximab, following the first intravenous dose. Therefore, in this trial, with PFS as the primary endpoint, a quadruplet, B-DRC was compared with a control arm of a modified DRC regimen. The investigators indicated that the increasing use of ibrutinib, a BTKi, substantially slowed the accrual rate, leading to the trial's premature closure. Overall, 204 patients were enrolled in the study for which the ORR at the end of treatment (six cycles) appeared comparable between the 2 groups: 95% for B-DRC versus 87% for DRC, $P = .07$; however, at the end of the 3 cycles, ORR and major responses were observed in a higher proportion of patients who were treated with B-DRC [ORR 79 versus 57%, and major response rate 65% versus 33%, $P < .01$]. Ultimately, as the best response, the MRR of 85% and 82% were attained with B-DRC and DRC, respectively, $P = .60$. A numerically higher proportion of patients who were treated with B-DRC achieved a deeper response (very good partial response [VGPR] or better rates 33% vs 21%). The responses were attained faster in patients on B-DRC (median time-to-first response for B-DRC was 3.0 vs 5.5 months for DRC]) Importantly, no difference in the 2-year PFS rates was noted between the 2 arms (81% with B-DRC vs 73% with DRC $P = .32$). The PFS rate was similar to the 2-year PFS rate of 67% achieved with the classic DRC regimen, and the rates of peripheral neuropathy, as expected, were higher with B-DRC (18% vs 3%).[13,14] Although the addition of bortezomib to DRC could hasten the attainment of deeper remission among patients in need of a rapid response, these data primarily confirmed that DRC remains an attractive triplet for patients with WM, with a more acceptable toxicity profile, and minimal lymphopenia (3%–5% vs >50% with BR) a factor that may play a role in selecting bridging therapy options in the era of chimeric antigen receptor (CAR) T-cells-based approaches that are being evaluated in patients with relapsed and/or refractory WM.[15]

Bendamustine exhibits the characteristics of an alkylating agent and a purine nucleoside with a favorable toxicity profile. Bendamustine-rituximab (BR) became one of the widely adopted frontline CIT regimens for WM following the results of the StiLNHL1-2003 trial, a landmark phase 3 randomized controlled, noninferiority study that compared bendamustine and rituximab versus R-CHOP in 447 patients with mantle-cell lymphoma and indolent lymphomas, including a subset of 41 patients with LPL/WM.[16] The subset analysis reported a longer PFS with BR (69.5 months compared with 28.1 months; hazard ratio [HR] 0.33, P = .003) with R-CHOP, despite equally high ORR in both arms (96% with BR and 94% with R-CHOP) among patients with previously untreated WM. Neither regimen was successful in inducing CRs, and OS rates were similar at the time of the last report, although the sub-performance of the control (R-CHOP) arm in this study with respect to the PFS endpoint compared with the R-CHOP arm of the GLSG trial was noteworthy.[7] Along with the StiLNHL1-2003 trial data, the BRIGHT trial comparing BR versus R-CHOP/R-CVP in indolent lymphomas confirmed the superiority of BR on PFS (5-year PFS rate of 65% vs 56%, HR 0.6, P = .002). Only 11 out of the 447 patients had a diagnosis of LPL/WM in this study.[17,18] However, it was the subsequent larger, StiLNHL7-2008 trial involving 296 patients that reaffirmed the remarkable efficacy of BR induction, although its primary objective was to assess the role of rituximab maintenance among the newly diagnosed patients with active WM who had achieved at least a PR to 6 cycles of BR plus 2 additional cycles of rituximab.[16,19] The median PFS with BR induction alone was 69 months, almost identical to the findings of the preceding StiLNHL1-2003 trial (median PFS 69.5 months, **Table 1**).[16,19] Only 7 cases of second myeloid malignancies were noted in both BR and R-CHOP groups among 447 patients despite a long median follow-up of almost 10 years.[20] The patients in the maintenance arm received rituximab every 2 months for 2 years.[20] Among patients achieving at least a PR to BR, the median PFS was 101 months in the rituximab maintenance cohort versus 83 months in the BR alone cohort, but this difference in outcome was not statistically significant (HR 0.80; P = .32). The study results have not been published yet but the most recent update in 2022 demonstrated the median PFS of 118 months with maintenance compared with 106 months patients in the rituximab maintenance arm following BR induction, P = .27, after 118 months of follow-up.[16,21] The OS rates were also similar, contradicting the data from retrospective studies suggesting the benefit of using rituximab maintenance therapy among the responders.[22,23] However, a subset of patients above the age of 65 showed significantly longer PFS with maintenance in an unplanned posthoc analysis of the StiLNHL7-2008 trial, suggesting there might be a benefit of maintenance therapy in elderly patients. This issue can only be settled with prospective studies in specific subsets of patients. Additionally, the StiLNHL7-2008 demonstrated that the progression within 24 months of initiation of BR portended dismal survival, underscoring the need to develop novel targeted therapies for this subset of patients.[24]

A major adverse effect of BR is myelosuppression, in addition to lymphodepletion. In the StiLNHL1-2003 and BRIGHT trials, respectively, grade 3/4 lymphopenia was reported in 62% to 74% of patients treated with BR as compared with 30% to 43% of patients in the control arm.[16,17] Importantly, alopecia is not observed with BR (0% in the StiLNHL1 trial), and the rates of paresthesias are markedly lower than R-CHOP. However, cutaneous adverse events, such as erythema (16% vs 9%) and allergic skin reaction (15% vs 6%) were higher with BR than R-CHOP.[16] Second myeloid malignancies are an important concern when treating patients with CIT. In the most recent update of the StiL trial, after 86 months of follow-up, 1 of 296 patients treated with BR developed myelodysplastic syndrome and none had acute leukemia.[21] Another retrospective study, with a 9-year median follow-up, reported 0.5% per-person per-year of developing MDS or AML which translated to a cumulative incidence of 6% after treatment

Table 1
Results from clinical trials with chemoimmunotherapy as frontline treatment in Waldenström macroglobulinemia

Regimen	Study	Phase	N (TN)	ORR (%)	MRR %	CR%/VGPR%	PFS (m)[a]	OS (m)[a]	Comments
Dexamethasone/Rituximab/Cyclophosphamide (DRC)[10,11,14]	Kastritis et al,[10] 2015	II	72	83	74	7	35	95	A well-tolerated, 21-d moderately effective regimen.
	Buske et al,[1] 2021	II	96	91	82	1/20	73% at 2 y	Not reached at 2 y	Six 28-d cycles of DRC regimen using SQ rituximab from C2-C6 shows similar 2-y PFS to the 6 courses of the original 21-d C.
Rituximab/Bendamustine (BR)[16,24]	StiLNHL1-2003	III (subgroup analysis of WM cohort)	41	96	96	0	69.5		Although PFS of BR was markedly higher than that of R-CHOP (control arm, median 28 m), no OS difference was noted at 45m of follow up
	StiL NHL7-2008 MAINTAIN trial	III	266	93	88	1/24	69	NR	Adding rituximab maintenance post-BR (x 6C)+ R (x 2C) among pts with ≥PR did not statistically improve PFS or OS.
Bortezomib/Dex/Rituximab/Cyclophosphamide (B-DRC)[14]	Buske et al,[7] 2009	II	96	95	85	5/27	81% at 2 y	Not reached at 2y	Adding bortezomib to DRC showed no net PFS benefit against the DRC control. B-DRC increased the risk of neurotoxicity, but the time to deeper responses was shorter.
Lenalidomide/Rituximab/Cyclophosphamide/Dex (L-RCD)[12]	Rosenthal et al,[12] 2017	II	15	80	80	7	38	Not reached at 23 mo	Grade ≥3 neutropenia was observed in 42% of patients.

Regimen	Study	Phase							Comments
Fludarabine/Rituximab (FR)[47]	Treon et al,[36] 2011	II	27	96	89	5[d]/33	78[b]	Not reported	Pneumocystis carinii pneumonia and second myeloid malignancies, and disease transformation to aggressive lymphoma is a concern.
Rituximab/Cladribine (R-2CDA)[49]	Laszlo et al,[48] 2010	II	16	94	79	24[d]	Not reached[c]	93% at 43 mo follow-up.	No major infections were observed despite the lack of antimicrobial prophylaxis. No disease transformation was noted at 43 mo follow-up.
Fludarabine/Cyclophosphamide/Rituximab (FCR)[50]	Auer et al,[49] 2016 R2W	II	17	82	77	0/18	Not reached at 18 mo	88% at 18m	Grade ≥3 hematologic toxicities were higher with FCR compared to BCR
Bortezomib/Cyclophosphamide/Rituximab (BCR)[62]	Auer et al,[49] 2016 R2W	II	42	98	79	1/19	Not reached at 18 mo	98% at 18m	No grade 3 or higher neuropathy was reported.
Pentostatin/Cyclophosphamide ± Rituximab (PCR)[62,63]	Hensel et al,[61] 2005	II	9	77[d]	62[d]	15[d]	Not reported	Not reported	ORR was higher when R added to PC.
	Herth et al,[62] 2015	II	21	88[d]	68[d]	0/16[d]	84% at 2 y[d]	100% at 2 y[d]	Another small study showing the efficacy and safety of the adenosine deaminase inhibitor, pentostatin, combination therapy.

Results are reported for the treatment naïve subset only for studies that include relapsed/refractory patients in addition to the treatment naïve patients.

Abbreviations: BCR, bortezomib, cyclophosphamide, and dexamethasone; B-DRC, bortezomib, dexamethasone, rituximab, and cyclophosphamide; BR, bendamustine and rituximab; C, cycle; FR, fludarabine and rituximab; m, months; MRR, major response rate; ORR, overall response rate; OS, overall survival; PFS, progression-free survival; PR, partial response; pts, patients; R-2CDA, rituximab and cladribine, R, rituximab; y, years.

[a] Median unless specified.

[b] Time to progression (TTP).

[c] Time-to-treatment failure (TTF).

[d] For treatment-naïve and relapsed/refractory patients combined.

with bendamustine in patients with non-Hodgkin lymphoma.[25] Following the release of the StiLNHL1-2003 trial results, the remarkable efficacy and the relatively manageable toxicity profile of the BR doublet have been confirmed by other groups.[26–29]

In the French Innovative Leukemia Organization (FILO) multicenter, retrospective study involving 69 patients between 45 and 88 years of age (median 69 years), all patients except one achieved minor response or better, leading to an ORR of 97% with BR; the major response rate was 96%, with 19% attaining CR and 56% achieving VGPR or better.[29] The responses continued to deepen over 18 months, with cumulative ORR rates improving from 70% at 3 months, 91% at 6 months, to 97% at 18 months.[29] Thirty (44%) patients required either a dose reduction of bendamustine or a shorter course of BR, that is, fewer than 6 cycles. In the most recent update of this study, after a median follow-up of 68.5 months, the median OS was not reached, and the median PFS was 82 months (range: 75-NR). The 2-year rates of PFS and OS were remarkably high at 87% and 97%, respectively. Patients who received an abbreviated course had comparable PFS rates, consistent with the findings of a few other retrospective studies suggesting equivalent outcomes with 4 versus 6 cycles of BR. However, the UK group recently demonstrated inferior PFS in patients who received a lower cumulative dose of bendamustine during induction suggesting that 4 cycles might be insufficient.[30] In the FILO study, neither the presence of $MYD88^{mut}$ nor $CXCR4^{mut}$ impacted the response to BR. About one-half of the patients had prolonged cytopenias and 2 patients had treatment-related myeloid neoplasms.[28,29]

In a recent international collaborative effort, 208 patients who had received BR induction without rituximab maintenance were analyzed. After a median follow-up of 4 years, the estimated median PFS was approximately 70 months, mirroring the data generated by the STiL trials. The small subcohort of patients (11%) who had progression of disease (POD) within 24 months of BR therapy demonstrated shorter OS (5-year OS rate, 75% vs 94% for the rest, $P = .03$). This study also confirmed that BR was active irrespective of the $MYD88$ mutation status (4-year PFS rate was 71%). Among the small subset of patients (n = 48; 23%) in whom $CXCR4$ mutation status was available, 28% exhibited $CXCR4$ mutation, with a trend toward shorter PFS (median PFS 3.9 years vs 5.5 years for the subgroup with $CXCR4^{WT}$ genotype, $P = .056$), hinting at the possibility of $CXCR4$ mutations adversely affecting the outcome of patients on CIT as well, similar to the observations made with BTKi-based therapies.[31]

A Mayo Clinic study comparing BR (n = 83) to DRC (n = 92) and BDR (n = 45) demonstrated superior ORR with BR (98% vs 78% with DRC and 84% with BDR; $P = .003$) in the frontline setting. The median PFS was also superior with BR (median 5.2 years with BR vs 4.3 for DRC vs 1.8 years for BDR; $P < .001$), though no difference in the OS was observed among the 3 cohorts. Notably, the PFS with BDR was significantly shorter than the previously published reports in clinical trials with this regimen. Notably, the response rates for BR, DRC, or BDR regimens were not affected by the $MYD88$ mutation status, but the study did not address the impact of $CXCR4$ mutation on the different CITs.[32] The superiority of BR compared with other CIT regimens has also been demonstrated in a retrospective study by the DFCI Group and the WhiM-SICAL, a global patient-derived data registry for WM.[33,34]

An important retrospective, multicenter international collaborative study compared the outcomes of patients with treatment-naïve WM who were administered either BR or ibrutinib as primary therapy. The study excluded patients who received rituximab maintenance therapy and those with the $MYD88^{WT}$ genotype. In this analysis of age-matched patients, after a median follow-up of 4.2 years, the PFS rates were similar among the 2 treatment groups; 4-year PFS was 72% and 78% with BR and ibrutinib, respectively, $P = .14$. There was no OS difference between the 2 cohorts.

However, despite similar PFS and OS, the CR rates were substantially higher with BR (20% as compared with 2%, p=<0.001) as were the rates of VGPR or deeper response (50 vs 33% P = .009).[33] The WhiMSICAL global registry reported substantially longer time-to-next therapy with BR (n = 74) compared with BTK inhibitors (n = 23) in the frontline setting. Still, the baseline characteristics, including patient genotype, were unavailable in this analysis that was reliant on patient-reported rather than formally documented data.[35]

Another retrospective multicenter, international collaborative study reported the outcomes of 319 treatment-naive patients who were administered fixed-duration or Bortezomib, Dexamethasone, Rituximab (BDR), or a CIT (either BR or DRC). Importantly, this study identified that the depth of response to fixed-duration treatment was associated with prognosis. In the multivariate analysis, attaining a major response was independently associated with better PFS (HR 0.33, P < .001), time-to-next therapy (TTNT; HR 0.23, P < .001), and OS; (HR 0.31; P = .001) compared with patients who achieved less than a major response at the 6-month landmark from the commencement of fixed-duration treatment.[26]

The scant data with BR that are available for the relapsed and/or refractory (RR) setting are less impressive than the data in the frontline setting.[33,35,36] In a small phase 2 trial involving 30 patients with RRWM who were initially treated with BR, the median number of prior therapies was 2 (range 1–9), the ORR was 83%, VGPR and PR rates were 17% and 67%, respectively.[27] However, the median estimated time-to-progression (TTP) was 13 months, with protracted myelosuppression among patients previously exposed to purine analogs. One patient previously exposed to fludarabine and rituximab, and cyclophosphamide, prednisone, and rituximab developed MDS.[27] In a larger study of 71 patients with RRWM, after a median of 2 lines of therapy (most patients were exposed to alkylators and rituximab), ORR and major response rate were 80% and 75%, respectively, the CR rates were low at 7%. The quality of response was superior with the 90 mg/m2 dose of bendamustine. No cases of IgM flare were reported and among patients with high IgM levels, the initial infusion was postponed preventing hyperviscosity syndrome. The PFS rates were approximately 60% at 2 years, in contrast with 87% at 2 years in the treatment-naïve population in the FILO study. No patients developed a myeloid malignancy, but the follow-up was only 19 months.[37] These results suggest that maximal benefit, with a long treatment-free interval, is likely associated with using BR as primary rather than salvage therapy.

PURINE-ANALOG BASED REGIMENS

Purine/Nucleoside analogs, fludarabine, and cladribine (2-CDA), have a long track record in WM, with extensive data generated over the years in the frontline and salvage setting. The overall response rates as primary therapies are somewhat higher (40%–90% vs 3%–50% in RR setting).

Purine analogs can incorporate into the DNA and RNA strands and rapidly inhibit DNA replication plus gene transcription, affecting both the dividing and nondividing cells. Often irreversible, the major neurotoxicities (seizures, optic neuritis, cortical blindness, confusion) were not encountered with the lower doses of fludarabine used in lymphoproliferative disorders. In 1990, fludarabine was first used in 10 patients with RR and one with TN WM, with a single patient in the frontline setting and 40% in the relapsed-refractory setting achieving at least a partial response.[38] It has subsequently been studied extensively both as monotherapy as well as in combination with other agents, including alkylators and CD20 monoclonal antibodies, rituximab, and ofatumumab.[39–43]

It has not been directly compared with the other commonly used purine analog cladribine, but their tolerability and efficacy appear to be comparable.

Although it is only available as an intravenous formulation in the US, in a large, multicentric European phase 3 trial, oral fludarabine was compared with oral chlorambucil as primary therapy in 339 patients with WM (**Table 2**). Superior outcomes, including longer OS, were observed in the fludarabine arm. The study highlighted how the natural history of even an indolent lymphoma such as WM, with a relapsing-remitting course, could be determined by the choice of the initial therapy.[40] However, eventually, the case for its use in the frontline setting remained weak, given the associated toxicities, including prolonged myelosuppression (neutropenia and thrombocytopenia), increased risk of opportunistic infections, stem cell damage potentially adversely affecting stem cell mobilization for autologous transplantation, and the risk of histologic transformation as well as treatment-related myeloid malignancies.

Several combination therapies have also been evaluated; in particular, when combined with cyclophosphamide, a synergistic action has been observed as the cyclophosphamide-induced DNA breaks remain unrepaired in the presence of fludarabine. Tamburini and colleagues examined fludarabine plus cyclophosphamide (FC) involving 49 patients, 35 previously treated. An ORR was noted in 78% of the patients and the median TTF was 27 months. Notably, the responses with fludarabine may be delayed (median time of 10.8 months) and may continue to deepen even after the completion of treatment, similar to the observation made with several non-purine analog-based CIT regimens.[44,45] In vitro data also suggested synergistic activity with rituximab. Rituximab enhances cytotoxicity by fludarabine which also reciprocally, through the reduction of CD55 and CD59 expression on lymphocytes, increases their sensitivity to antibody-mediated apoptosis through caspase 3 and caspase 9 activation.[46] Consequently, better quality of responses and more durable responses are observed when fludarabine is combined with immunochemotherapy. In the study by Treon and colleagues, evaluating the fludarabine-rituximab combination in 43 patients of whom 27 (63%) were treatment-naïve, the ORR and MRR were 95%, and 86%, respectively.[47] After a median follow-up of 40.3 months, the median estimated time-to-progression (TTP) for the entire cohort was 51.2 months. It was significantly shorter in patients who received fludarabine and rituximab (FR) in the salvage setting (estimated 38 months) compared with FR as primary therapy (estimated 78 months). In this study, 7% of patients transformed to aggressive lymphoma. In comparison, another 7% of patients had developed AML/MDS at a median time of 21 months and 39 months, respectively, from the initiation of FR.[47]

Tedeschi and colleagues examined 6 cycles of the FCR (fludarabine, cyclophosphamide, and rituximab) regimen in patients with RRWM (n = 57) and TN with WM (n = 25). The ORR was 88%, with an MRR of 64% at treatment discontinuation, which improved to 76% at the best response. The PFS and OS rates were the same at 96% for 3 years. In a multivariate analysis, only the TN status before FCR (median PFS: 79 months for patients with RR, vs not reached; $P = .02$) and age (median PFS 46 months for patients over 65, vs not reached; $P = .006$) significantly impacted PFS.[48] Laszlo and colleagues evaluated subcutaneous cladribine with rituximab in patients with TN and RR. A high ORR of 90% was observed.[49] Clinicians should remain vigilant to additional supportive care, including growth factor support, Pneumocystis jiroveci, and herpes prophylaxis that patients may require on purine analog combinations, particularly those who are heavily pretreated.

The NCT01592981 (R2W) trial, is a non-comparative phase 2 study, with a primary endpoint of ORR. The trial randomly assigned 60 treatment-naïve patients in a 2:1 fashion to either subcutaneous bortezomib, oral cyclophosphamide, and intravenous

Table 2
Results from clinical trials of chemotherapy alone (without immunotherapy) in Waldenström macroglobulinemia

Study	Phase	Treatment	Patients (n)	ORR/MRR (%)	CR (%)	PFS[a] and/or OS
Dimopoulos et al,[38] 1993	II	Fludarabine	2, TN; 26, RR	100 (TN), 31 (RR)/36[b]	4	DOR (median): 38 mo[b]; OS (median): 32 mo[b]
Leblond et al,[39] 2009	III	Fludarabine vs chlorambucil	339, TN	46 vs 36/ - vs -	-	PFS (median): 37.8 mo vs 27.1 mo; OS (median): NR vs 69.8 mo
Foran et al,[40] 1999	II	Fludarabine	19, TN	79/79	5	PFS (median): 3.4 y; OS (median): NR
Dhodapkar et al,[41] 2001 S9003.	II	Fludarabine	118, TN; 64, RR	38/23	3	5-y PFS: 62% (TN), 36% (RR); 5-y OS: 49% (TN), 30% (RR)
Tamburini et al,[44] 2005	II	FC	14, TN; 35, RR	85/-	-	TTF (median)[b]: 27 mo; OS (median)[b]: NR
Dimopoulos et al,[63] 2003	II	FC	2, TN; 9, RR	55[b]/55[b]	-	PFS (median): 24 mo[b]; OS at 2 y: 70%[b]
Kyle et al,[64] 2000	II	Chlorambucil	46, TN	70/-	-	OS (median): 5.4 y

Abbreviations: DOR, duration-of-response; FC, fludarabine and cyclophosphamide; MRR, major response rate; not reported; NR, not reached; ORR, overall response rate; OS, overall survival; PFS, progression-free survival; RR, relapsed and/or refractory; TN, treatment-naïve; TTF, time-to-treatment failure.
[a] Some studies may have reported DOR or TTF instead of PFS.
[b] Responses for patients with TN and RR combined.

rituximab (BCR) or FCR for 6 cycles. It showed an ORR of 98% and 79% and MRR of 82% and 77%, respectively, with BCR and FCR.[50] The reduced rates and absence of grade 3 or higher of treatment-emergent peripheral neuropathy in the BCR arm were ascribed to the change in the route (from intravenous to subcutaneous) and frequency (from twice weekly to weekly) of bortezomib administration. After 18 months of follow-up, 3 patients in the BCR arm had progressed but none in the FCR arm (n = 17). However, despite the short follow-up, three deaths were reported: one from pneumonia in the BCR arm and 2 MDS-related in the FCR arm. No cases of MDS were observed in the BCR arm. The final results of this trial are awaited.[50]

Given the associated toxicities and the availability of equally, if not more effective therapies, purine analogs are used only in patients with RR disease when safer, effective alternatives are unavailable.

IMPACT OF UNDERLYING WALDENSTRÖM MACROGLOBULINEMIA-RELATED SOMATIC MUTATIONS ON PATIENT OUTCOMES WITH CHEMOIMMUNOTHERAPY

Studies have identified that $MYD88^{WT}$ WM is associated with a higher risk of histologic transformation to an aggressive lymphoma and the progression of smoldering WM to active disease.[51,52] Unlike the observation made with ibrutinib, the first-generation BTKi, within the sparsely available data, the patients' $MYD88$ genotype does not impact CIT-treated patients' outcomes. Compared with $CXCR4^{WT}$, a concurrent alteration in $CXCR4$ with $MYD88^{mut}$ confers an inferior response to BTKi-based therapy but its impact on the response to CIT is not well studied. $CXCR4^{WHIM/NS}$ mutations in smoldering WM may also be associated with a shorter treatment initiation time but do not appear to impact OS so far.[53,54] A recent multi-institutional collaborative effort, however, showed a trend toward inferior response and shorter PFS in patients that harbored $CXCR4$ mutations compared with those that exhibited $CXCR4^{WT}$ genotype on BR primary therapy.[31] The mutational data for $MYD88$ and $CXCR4$ genes have helped pave the way for personalized treatment for WM, especially about ibrutinib monotherapy. Still, their impact on outcomes with conventional CIT remains to be fully elucidated. Additionally, generally a marker of poor prognosis, how the varying proportions of $TP53$ alterations reported in WM by the recent next-generation sequencing-based studies impact the outcome of patients treated with CIT is not yet well studied.[55–58]

The Case for Chemoimmunotherapy Use in the Frontline Setting

Despite the emergence of multiple effective treatments in the frontline setting for patients with WM, only some randomized trials have established the superiority of one regimen over the other. Various factors impact the decision-making for optimal frontline therapy, including the mutational profile, patient preference, performance status, and comorbidities.

In patients with TN symptomatic WM, we administer 6 cycles of BR without maintenance rituximab. This approach is effective even with $MYD88^{WT,}$ for which BTK inhibitors, particularly ibrutinib, have shown substantially reduced efficacy. Furthermore, among the BTK inhibitor-naïve patients, the efficacy of BTKi-based salvage regimens appears to remain uncompromised.

A fixed duration of treatment, achievement of deep and durable responses (median PFS of 5.5–6 years in all patients and nearly 9 years for patients who achieve at least a partial remission), along with the short-lived adverse effects that are manageable and predominantly confined to the 6-month duration of therapy are the major reasons for adopting BR as the primary regimen for WM. However, one should remain vigilant regarding the development of myeloid malignancies, prolonged lymphodepletion, and immunosuppression. In contrast to the incidence of the second myeloid malignancies (0.5% per person per year) with fixed-duration BR as salvage treatment, MDS and AML were exceedingly uncommon when BR was used as primary therapy for indolent lymphomas.[25,59] In patients with a serum IgM level of more than 4000 mg/dL, rituximab may be omitted from the initial couple of cycles of CIT to avoid an IgM flare that could worsen the symptoms of hyperviscosity, cryoglobulinemia or neuropathy.[60] In elderly patients above 70 years of age, we reduce the standard recommended dose of bendamustine from 90 mg/m^2 on days 1 and 2, to 70 mg/m^2/d over 2 days. For frail patients, DRC for six cycles is a viable alternative. While formal analyses have not been performed, limited duration BR is likely more cost-effective than continuous BTKi therapy.

Ongoing Studies with Chemoimmunotherapy as Primary Treatment

An ongoing single-arm, phase 2 Canadian study (NCT04624906, BRAWM) is assessing the efficacy of bendamustine and rituximab for six 28-day cycles concomitantly with the second-generation BTKi, acalabrutinib for an abbreviated duration of 1 year in previously untreated patients with WM. However, the primary study outcome measure is the rate of VGPR or deeper remission as the best response, the value of which as a surrogate for PFS and OS is unclear.

Another ongoing study (NCT05099471, VIVA-1), developed for previously untreated patients on the heels of the promising activity and tolerability of venetoclax monotherapy demonstrated among patients with RRWM,[61] is a phase 2, open-label, randomized trial designed to explore whether fixed-duration venetoclax plus rituximab combination increases the rate of CR/VGPR 12 months after randomization compared with DRC, irrespective of the patient genotype.

In summary, CIT is a highly effective approach for patients with WM. High-level evidence suggests that the choice of the initial regimen can potentially change the natural history of WM, a malignancy that remains incurable. True advances in the field would be made when substantial improvement over the high bar set by the BR therapy is overcome by other limited-duration regimens in the frontline setting, with minimal acute and long-term toxicities.

CLINICS CARE POINTS

- A phase 3 randomized controlled trial has shown higher efficacy and a more favorable toxicity profile of the bendamustine-rituximab (BR) compared with R-CHOP (rituximab, cyclophosphamide, doxorubicin, vincristine, and prednisone) among patients with treatment-naïve WM.
- High level evidence comparing BR and DRC regimens is absent.
- DRC appears to be inferior to BR in cross-trial comparisons and retrospective series involving treatment-naïve patients with WM.
- Purine analog-based CIT has been extensively evaluated in WM, although its use has waned, even in the multiply relapsed patient population, as effective and safer alternatives have emerged.

CONFLICT OF INTEREST

P. Kapoor is the principal investigator of trials for which Mayo Clinic has received research funding from Amgen, United States, Regeneron, United States, Bristol Myers

Squibb, United States, Loxo Pharmaceuticals, Ichnos, Karyopharm, Sanofi, United States, AbbVie and GlaxoSmithKline. P. Kapoor has served on the Advisory Boards of BeiGene, Pharmacyclics, X4 Pharmaceuticals, Kite, Oncopeptides, Angitia Bio, GlaxoSmithKline, AbbVie, and Sanofi. J. Paludo reports Honoraria to institution: Abbvie and research funding to institution: Karyopharm and Biofourmis. J. Abeykoon reports research funding from Qurient therapeutics.

REFERENCES

1. Buske C, Leblond V. Waldenstrom's macroglobulinemia. In: Dreyling M, Ladetto M, editors. Indolent lymphomas. New York: Springer; 2021. p. 143–61.

2. Sekhar J, et al. Waldenstrom macroglobulinemia: a Surveillance, Epidemiology, and End Results database review from 1988 to 2005. Leuk Lymphoma 2012; 53(8):1625–6.

3. Fonseca R, Hayman S. Waldenström macroglobulinaemia. Br J Haematol 2007; 138(6):700–20.

4. Morel P, Merlini G. Risk stratification in Waldenström macroglobulinemia. Expert Rev Hematol 2012;5(2):187–99.

5. Dimopoulos MA, et al. Predictive factors for response to rituximab in Waldenstrom's macroglobulinemia. Clin Lymphoma 2005;5(4):270–2.

6. Furman RR, et al. Once-weekly ofatumumab in untreated or relapsed Waldenström's macroglobulinaemia: an open-label, single-arm, phase 2 study. Lancet Haematol 2017;4(1):e24–34.

7. Buske C, et al. The addition of rituximab to front-line therapy with CHOP (R-CHOP) results in a higher response rate and longer time to treatment failure in patients with lymphoplasmacytic lymphoma: results of a randomized trial of the German Low-Grade Lymphoma Study Group (GLSG). Leukemia 2009;23(1): 153–61.

8. Abonour R, et al. Phase II Pilot Study of Rituximab + CHOP in Patients with Newly Diagnosed Waldenström's Macroglobulinemia, an Eastren Cooperative Oncology Group Trial (Study E1A02). Blood 2007;110(11):3616.

9. Okada N, et al. Risk Factors for Early-Onset Peripheral Neuropathy Caused by Vincristine in Patients With a First Administration of R-CHOP or R-CHOP-Like Chemotherapy. J Clin Med Res 2014;6(4):252–60.

10. Kastritis E, et al. Dexamethasone, rituximab, and cyclophosphamide as primary treatment of Waldenström macroglobulinemia: final analysis of a phase 2 study. Blood 2015;126(11):1392–4.

11. Dimopoulos MA, et al. Primary treatment of Waldenström macroglobulinemia with dexamethasone, rituximab, and cyclophosphamide. J Clin Oncol 2007;25(22): 3344–9.

12. Rosenthal A, et al. A phase 2 study of lenalidomide, rituximab, cyclophosphamide, and dexamethasone (LR-CD) for untreated low-grade non-Hodgkin lymphoma requiring therapy. Am J Hematol 2017;92(5):467–72.

13. Buske C, et al. Bortezomib in Combination with Dexamethasone, Rituximab and Cyclophosphamide (B-DRC) As First - Line Treatment of Waldenstrom's Macroglobulinemia: Results of a Prospectively Randomized Multicenter European Phase II Trial. Blood 2020;136(Supplement 1):26.

14. Buske C, et al. Bortezomib-Dexamethasone, Rituximab, and Cyclophosphamide as First-Line Treatment for Waldenström's Macroglobulinemia: A Prospectively Randomized Trial of the European Consortium for Waldenström's Macroglobulinemia. J Clin Oncol 2023;22:01805.

15. Saito H, et al. Prolonged lymphocytopenia after bendamustine therapy in patients with relapsed or refractory indolent B-cell and mantle cell lymphoma. Blood Cancer J 2015;5(10):e362.
16. Rummel MJ, et al. Bendamustine plus rituximab versus CHOP plus rituximab as first-line treatment for patients with indolent and mantle-cell lymphomas: an open-label, multicentre, randomised, phase 3 non-inferiority trial. Lancet (London, England) 2013;381(9873):1203–10.
17. Flinn IW, et al. First-Line Treatment of Patients With Indolent Non-Hodgkin Lymphoma or Mantle-Cell Lymphoma With Bendamustine Plus Rituximab Versus R-CHOP or R-CVP: Results of the BRIGHT 5-Year Follow-Up Study. J Clin Oncol 2019;37(12):984–91.
18. Flinn IW, et al. Randomized trial of bendamustine-rituximab or R-CHOP/R-CVP in first-line treatment of indolent NHL or MCL: the BRIGHT study. Blood 2014; 123(19):2944–52.
19. Rummel MJ, et al. Bendamustine Plus Rituximab Followed By Rituximab Maintenance for Patients with Untreated Advanced Follicular Lymphomas. Results from the StiL NHL 7-2008 Trial (MAINTAIN trial) (ClinicalTrials.gov Identifier: NCT00877214). Blood 2014;124(21):3052.
20. Rummel MJ, et al. Bendamustine plus rituximab (B-R) versus CHOP plus rituximab (CHOP-R) as first-line treatment in patients with indolent lymphomas: Nine-year updated results from the StiL NHL1 study. J Clin Oncol 2017;35(15_suppl):7501.
21. Rummel M. Bendamustine plus rituximab followed by rituximab maintenance for patients with untreated advanced follicular lymphomas. Results from the StiL NHL 7-2008 trial (MAINTAIN trial) (ClinicalTrials.gov identifier: NCT00877214). Madrid, Spain: IWWM-11 meeting; 2022.
22. Castillo JJ, et al. Response and survival for primary therapy combination regimens and maintenance rituximab in Waldenström macroglobulinaemia. Br J Haematol 2018;181(1):77–85.
23. Zanwar S, et al. Rituximab-based maintenance therapy in Waldenström macroglobulinemia: A case control study. J Clin Oncol 2019;37(15_suppl):7559.
24. Rummel MJ, et al. Two Years Rituximab Maintenance Vs. Observation after First Line Treatment with Bendamustine Plus Rituximab (B-R) in Patients with Waldenström's Macroglobulinemia (MW): Results of a Prospective, Randomized, Multicenter Phase 3 Study (the StiL NHL7-2008 MAINTAIN trial). Blood 2019; 134(Supplement_1):343.
25. Martin P, et al. Long-term outcomes, secondary malignancies and stem cell collection following bendamustine in patients with previously treated non-Hodgkin lymphoma. Br J Haematol 2017;178(2):250–6.
26. Paludo J, et al. Bendamustine and rituximab (BR) versus dexamethasone, rituximab, and cyclophosphamide (DRC) in patients with Waldenström macroglobulinemia. Ann Hematol 2018;97(8):1417–25.
27. Tedeschi A, et al. Bendamustine and rituximab combination is safe and effective as salvage regimen in Waldenström macroglobulinemia. Leuk Lymphoma 2015; 56(9):2637–42.
28. Laribi K, et al. Bendamustine plus rituximab in newly-diagnosed Waldenström macroglobulinaemia patients. A study on behalf of the French Innovative Leukaemia Organization (FILO). Br J Haematol 2019;186(1):146–9.
29. Laribi K, et al. Long-Term Follow-up of Bendamustine Plus Rituximab Regimen in 69 Treatment Naïve (TN) Patients with Waldenström Macroglobulinemia, a Study on Behalf of the French Innovative Leukemia Organization (FILO). Blood 2022; 140(Supplement 1):3627–8.

30. Arulogun SO, et al. Bendamustine Plus Rituximab for the Treatment of Waldenström Macroglobulinaemia: Patient Outcomes and Impact of Bendamustine Dosing. Blood 2020;136:10–1.
31. Zanwar S, et al. P1159: a multicenter, international collaborative study evaluating frontline therapy with bendamustine rituximab for Waldenström macroglobulinemia. HemaSphere 2022;6.
32. Abeykoon JP, et al. Assessment of fixed-duration therapies for treatment-naïve Waldenström macroglobulinemia. Am J Hematol 2021;96(8):945–53.
33. Tohidi-Esfahani I, et al. WhiMSICAL: A global Waldenström's Macroglobulinemia patient-derived data registry capturing treatment and quality of life outcomes. Am J Hematol 2021;96(6):E218–22.
34. Abeykoon JP, et al. Bendamustine rituximab (BR) versus ibrutinib (Ibr) as primary therapy for Waldenström macroglobulinemia (WM): An international collaborative study. J Clin Oncol 2022;40(16_suppl):7566.
35. Perera ND, et al. Prognostic impact of depth of response in Waldenström macroglobulinemia patients treated with fixed duration chemoimmunotherapy. J Clin Oncol 2021;39(15_suppl):8049.
36. Treon SP, et al. Bendamustine therapy in patients with relapsed or refractory Waldenström's macroglobulinemia. Clin Lymphoma Myeloma Leuk 2011;11(1):133–5.
37. Kantarjian HM, et al. Fludarabine therapy in macroglobulinemic lymphoma. Blood 1990;75(10):1928–31.
38. Dimopoulos MA, et al. Fludarabine therapy in Waldenström's macroglobulinemia. Am J Med 1993;95(1):49–52.
39. Leblond V, et al. Results of a randomized trial of chlorambucil versus fludarabine for patients with untreated Waldenström macroglobulinemia, marginal zone lymphoma, or lymphoplasmacytic lymphoma. J Clin Oncol 2013;31(3):301–7.
40. Foran JM, et al. Multicenter phase II study of fludarabine phosphate for patients with newly diagnosed lymphoplasmacytoid lymphoma, Waldenström's macroglobulinemia, and mantle-cell lymphoma. J Clin Oncol 1999;17(2):546–53.
41. Dhodapkar MV, et al. Prognostic factors and response to fludarabine therapy in patients with Waldenstrom macroglobulinemia: results of United States intergroup trial (Southwest Oncology Group S9003). Blood 2001;98(1):41–8.
42. Thalhammer-Scherrer R, et al. Fludarabine therapy in Waldenström's macroglobulinemia. Ann Hematol 2000;79(10):556–9.
43. Castillo JJ, et al. Deepening of response after completing rituximab-containing therapy in patients with Waldenstrom macroglobulinemia. Am J Hematol 2020;95(4):372–8.
44. Tamburini J, et al. Fludarabine plus cyclophosphamide in Waldenström's macroglobulinemia: results in 49 patients. Leukemia 2005;19(10):1831–4.
45. Furlan A, et al. Low-dose fludarabine increases rituximab cytotoxicity in B-CLL cells by triggering caspases activation in vitro. Leuk Lymphoma 2010;51(1):107–13.
46. Treon SP, et al. Long-term outcomes to fludarabine and rituximab in Waldenström macroglobulinemia. Blood 2009;113(16):3673–8.
47. Tedeschi A, et al. Fludarabine plus cyclophosphamide and rituximab in Waldenstrom macroglobulinemia: an effective but myelosuppressive regimen to be offered to patients with advanced disease. Cancer 2012;118(2):434–43.
48. Laszlo D, et al. Rituximab and subcutaneous 2-chloro-2'-deoxyadenosine combination treatment for patients with Waldenstrom macroglobulinemia: clinical and biologic results of a phase II multicenter study. J Clin Oncol 2010;28(13):2233–8.

49. Auer RL, et al. R2W: Subcutaneous Bortezomib, Cyclophosphamide and Rituximab (BCR) Versus Fludarabine, Cyclophosphamide and Rituximab (FCR) for Initial Therapy of WaldenströM's Macroglobulinemia: A Randomised Phase II Study. Blood 2016;128(22):618.
50. Abeykoon JP, et al. MYD88 mutation status does not impact overall survival in Waldenstrom macroglobulinemia. Am J Hematol 2018;93(2):187–94.
51. Zanwar S, et al. Impact of MYD88(L265P) mutation status on histological transformation of Waldenström Macroglobulinemia. Am J Hematol 2020;95(3):274–81.
52. Varettoni M, et al. Pattern of somatic mutations in patients with Waldenström macroglobulinemia or IgM monoclonal gammopathy of undetermined significance. Haematologica 2017;102(12):2077–85.
53. Poulain S, et al. Genomic Landscape of CXCR4 Mutations in Waldenstrom Macroglobulinemia. Clin Cancer Res 2016;22(6):1480–8.
54. Wang Y, et al. Molecular and genetic biomarkers implemented from next-generation sequencing provide treatment insights in clinical practice for Waldenström macroglobulinemia. Neoplasia 2021;23(4):361–74.
55. Christian A, et al. Importance of sequential analysis of TP53 variation in patients with Waldenström Macroglobulinaemia. Br J Haematol 2019;186(4):e73–6.
56. Gustine JN, et al. TP53 mutations are associated with mutated MYD88 and CXCR4, and confer an adverse outcome in Waldenström macroglobulinaemia. Br J Haematol 2019;184(2):242–5.
57. Poulain S, et al. TP53 Mutation and Its Prognostic Significance in Waldenstrom's Macroglobulinemia. Clin Cancer Res 2017;23(20):6325–35.
58. Penne M, et al. Extended Follow-up of Patients Treated With Bendamustine for Lymphoid Malignancies. Clin Lymphoma, Myeloma & Leukemia 2017;17(10):637–44.
59. Ghobrial IM, et al. Initial immunoglobulin M 'flare' after rituximab therapy in patients diagnosed with Waldenstrom macroglobulinemia: an Eastern Cooperative Oncology Group Study. Cancer 2004;101(11):2593–8.
60. Castillo JJ, et al. Venetoclax in Previously Treated Waldenström Macroglobulinemia. J Clin Oncol 2022;40(1):63–71.
61. Hensel M, et al. Pentostatin/Cyclophosphamide with or Without Rituximab: An Effective Regimen for Patients with Waldenström's Macroglobulinemia/Lymphoplasmacytic Lymphoma. Clinical Lymphoma and Myeloma 2005;6(2):131–5.
62. Herth I, et al. Pentostatin, cyclophosphamide and rituximab is a safe and effective treatment in patients with Waldenström's macroglobulinemia. Leuk Lymphoma 2015;56(1):97–102.
63. Dimopoulos MA, et al. Treatment of Waldenstrom's macroglobulinemia with the combination of fludarabine and cyclophosphamide. Leuk Lymphoma 2003;44(6):993–6.
64. Kyle RA, et al. Waldenström's macroglobulinaemia: a prospective study comparing daily with intermittent oral chlorambucil. Br J Haematol 2000;108(4):737–42.

Proteasome Inhibitor-Based Regimens in the Frontline Management of Waldenström Macroglobulinemia

Eirini Solia, MD, Meletios A. Dimopoulos, MD,
Efstathios Kastritis, MD*

KEYWORDS

- Bortezomib • Carfilzomib • Ixazomib • First-line therapy • Neuropathy

KEY POINTS

- Proteasome inhibitors (PIs) remain an active treatment option for the frontline management of Waldenström Macroglobulinemia (WM).
- Bortezomib is effective either as a single agent or in combination with other regimens with high response rates observed in most studies, but neurotoxicity remains a major concern.
- Second-generation PIs, such as carfilzomib and ixazomib, provide active and neuropathy-sparing options, although with a different toxicity profile than bortezomib.
- The choice of each PI in the treatment of WM should be individualized owing to the heterogeneity of the disease's presentation and based on each patient's unique characteristics.

INTRODUCTION

Since the Swedish physician Jan G. Waldenström described for the first time what is now Waldenström Macroglobulinemia (WM) in 1944,[1] the approach to therapy for the disease has made substantial progress. WM is a rare B-cell non-Hodgkin lymphoma characterized by the infiltration of the bone marrow by clonal lymphoplasmacytic cells leading to monoclonal immunoglobulin M (IgM) production.[2,3] WM accounts for only 1% to 2% of all hematologic malignancies with a 2-to-1 male predominance[4] but has a heterogeneous clinical presentation with clinical features of symptomatic disease that include cytopenias, most commonly anemia, hepatomegaly, splenomegaly, lymphadenopathy, fatigue and other B symptoms, IgM-related disorders, such as hyperviscosity-related symptoms, peripheral neuropathies, cryoglobulinemia, cold

Department of Clinical Therapeutics, National and Kapodistrian University of Athens, Athens, Greece
* Corresponding author. 80 Vas. Sofia Avenue & Lourou Street, Athens 11528, Greece.
E-mail addresses: ekastritis@med.uoa.gr; ekastritis@gmail.com

Hematol Oncol Clin N Am 37 (2023) 689–705
https://doi.org/10.1016/j.hoc.2023.04.004
0889-8588/23/© 2023 Elsevier Inc. All rights reserved.

hemonc.theclinics.com

agglutinin-related symptoms, and light chain amyloidosis.[1,5] Most patients with WM (>90%) carry a somatic mutation in the MYD88 gene (MYD88[L265P]). In comparison, mutations in the CXCR4 gene are observed in 30% to 40% of patients and are related to increased levels of IgM and risk of hyperviscosity as well as shorter disease remissions in patients treated with Bruton Tyrosine Kinase inhibitors (BTKis).[6]

WM is considered an incurable disease and, for symptomatic patients with WM treatment, one needs to consider a variety of disease-related complications and therapy-related toxicities, especially for older patients. Today, immunotherapy combinations targeting anti-CD20 (mainly rituximab) with chemotherapy (such as the DRC and BR combinations) remain widely used in everyday clinical practice. However, the introduction of BTKis has offered another very effective treatment option.[7–10] Proteasome inhibitors (PIs), first approved in myeloma, have also shown activity in WM, been used in combination regimens for the treatment of symptomatic newly diagnosed or relapsed/refractory WM, and have also become an essential part of chemotherapy-free regimens. PIs have been explored in several single-arm phase 2 studies and recently in a randomized phase 2 study. This review aims to present the current data on the efficacy of PIs, their toxicity profile, and their role in managing previously untreated patients with WM in the context of currently available options.

PROTEASOME INHIBITORS
Mechanisms of Action

The ubiquitin-proteasome pathway has a key role in the degradation of various proteins, including ubiquitinated proteins. This process is vital for the function and homeostasis of the cells, and its deregulation may affect cancer cells. From that point of view, the proteasome plays an important role in cellular homeostasis and is a target against cancer cells.[11] The 26S proteasome is present in the cytoplasm and nucleus and includes two 19S regulatory complexes and a 20S core composed of 4 rings (2 α and 2 β rings).[12] Each β ring consists of 7 subunits, including 3 sites: a caspase-like site, a trypsin-like site, and a chymotrypsin-like site, which has the most proteolytic ability. The 19S complex identifies the protein that will be degraded and deubiquitinated. PIs are categorized into 5 groups: peptide aldehydes, peptide vinyl sulfones, peptide boronates, peptide epoxyketones, and β-lactones.[13] Different PIs have different affinities for the proteasome catalytic subunits and may be reversible or irreversible inhibitors. For instance, bortezomib is a boronic acid dipeptide that inhibits 26S proteasome reversibly, whereas carfilzomib is a tetrapeptide epoxyketone, an analogue of epoxomicin, and inhibits 20S proteasome irreversibly.[14–16] PIs inhibit the degradation of ubiquitinated proteins by the proteasome, leading to the accumulation of the ubiquitinated proteins and an increase in the stress of the endoplasmic reticulum (ER). The unfolded proteins trigger a signaling pathway, the unfolded protein response (UPR), a stress response. UPR assists cells in handling the increased number of unfolded proteins. An excessive stress UPR can lead to apoptosis.[13,17–19]

Bortezomib in Waldenström Macroglobulinemia

Bortezomib is a dipeptide boronic derivative acid that reversibly inhibits the 26S proteasome. As a result of its inhibitory activity in the proteasome, it induces ER stress-promoting apoptosis.[19,20] Bortezomib is effective and has been approved for treating multiple myeloma (MM) and mantle cell lymphoma. However, the main adverse effect of bortezomib is neurotoxicity, which is not a class effect. The neurotoxicity is mostly reversible, at least to a significant degree, and seems less frequent and severe with dose modifications (weekly instead of twice a week) and subcutaneous (SC; compared with intravenous [IV]) administration.

Bortezomib has been tested in clinical trials as a single agent or in combination with other regimens in the first-line therapy in patients with WM. The results of the published studies are summarized in **Table 1**.

As a single agent for treatment-naïve patients, bortezomib has been tested as part of 2 clinical trials that included mostly patients with relapsed or refractory WM, and generally in small numbers of patients. Chen and colleagues[21] ran a phase 2 multicenter study and observed that the response rates were similar between treatment-naïve and pretreated patients, 3 out of 12 (25%) and 4 out of 15 (27%), respectively. Neurotoxicity, especially sensory neuropathy, was a frequent adverse event, but overall, the drug was well tolerated. Similar toxicity was described in the majority of enrolled patients, one of whom was previously untreated, in the multicenter study of Treon and colleagues.[22]

Bortezomib has been extensively investigated with other agents, including several studies for treating newly diagnosed symptomatic WM. Ghobrial and colleagues,[23] in a phase 2 study, enrolled 26 untreated patients with WM who received bortezomib and rituximab (VR). Bortezomib was given weekly every 28 days for 6 cycles without maintenance therapy. The overall response rate (ORR) was 88% (in 23/26 patients), whereas major responses (major response rate [MRR]) were observed in 17 (65%) patients. The median time to progression (mTTP) at the time of the study was not reached, and the estimated 1-year event-free survival (EFS) rate was 79%. The long-term results of this study revealed that in a total of 63 patients, including previously untreated (26/63) and pretreated (37/63) ones, the mTTP and median duration of response (DOR) were 1.6 (1.1–5) and 1.4 (0.6–5) years, respectively.[24] The most frequent grade 3 and 4 adverse events were neutropenia, anemia, and thrombocytopenia, but no grade 3 neuropathy was reported. Sensory neuropathy grade 1 to 2 was observed in 14 patients (54%).[23] The updated study confirmed the previous results, suggesting serious adverse events owing to hematological complications in 10 of 63 enrolled patients, previously treated and untreated. Other most common no serious adverse events included fatigue and anemia.[24]

In another study, Zhang and colleagues[25] evaluated bortezomib with dexamethasone in untreated Chinese patients with WM. Considering bortezomib's neurotoxicity, they administered it at a lower dose (1 mg/m^2). The ORR reached 80%, and at a median follow-up time of 36 months, all patients were alive, and 6 (60%) did not have disease progression. The most frequent toxicity was low-grade (G1–2) neuropathy that did not lead to the discontinuation of bortezomib.

The most investigated combination is the chemotherapy-free regimen of bortezomib with rituximab and dexamethasone (BDR). Treon and colleagues[26] tested BDR in 23 previously untreated symptomatic patients with WM. Bortezomib was administered IV at a dose of 1.3 mg/m^2 on days 1, 4, 8, and 11, every 21 days for 4 cycles, followed by a maintenance phase. The ORR was 96%, and 19 patients (83%) achieved MRR. Two patients experienced an "IgM flare" and underwent plasmapheresis. Moreover, the median time to response (mTTR) was 1.4 months. The most common toxicities included peripheral neuropathy grade 2 to 3, anemia, infections without neutropenia, and thrombocytopenia. Notably, herpes zoster reactivation was observed in 4 of the first 7 patients, none receiving antiviral prophylaxis. Herpes zoster prophylaxis is now routinely recommended when bortezomib is used, and especially when corticosteroids are added, with or without rituximab, because of the increased risk of the virus reactivation.[26] The long-term outcomes of this study confirmed the high response rates (96% ORR and 91% MRR), and at a median

Table 1
Clinical studies of bortezomib in previously untreated patients with Waldenström macroglobulinemia

Study	Type of Study	Regimen	Dose and Schedule of PI	No of Untreated pts	Mutation	Results	Adverse Events of PI
Chen et al,[21] 2007	Multicenter phase 2 study trial	Bortezomib	1.3 mg/m^2 IV on d 1, 4, 8, 11 on a 21-d cycle for a median 6 cycles	12/27 (44%)	NA	Response rates: 3/12 (25%)	Anemia, neuropathy, Fatigue, nausea, neutropenia, thrombocytopenia[a]
Treon et al,[22] 2007	Multicenter phase 2 study	Bortezomib	1.3 mg/m^2 on d 1, 4, 8, and 11 Median no of cycles: 6	1/27	NA	For all pts: 27 (85.2%) ORR,[a] 13 (48.1%) MRR[a]	Sensory neuropathy, leukopenia, neutropenia, fatigue[a]
Ghobrial et al,[23] 2010	Phase 2 trial	VR	V: 1.6 mg/m^2 IV on d 1, 8, 15, every 28 d for 6 cycles R: 375 mg/m^2 per week in cycles 1 and 4	26 symptomatic	NA	23 (88%) ORR, 17 (65%) MRR, 1 (4%) CR, 1 (4%) nCR, 15 (58%) PR, 6 (23%) MR, 3 (12%) SD m f/u: 14 mo mDOR: NR, mPFS: NR, estimated 1-y PFS: 75%, mTTP: NR, estimated 1-y EFS: 79%, mOS: NR, estimated 1-y OS: 96% mTTNT: NR	G1 (n = 6, 23%), G2 (n = 10, 38%), G3 (n = 7, 27%), G4 (n = 3, 12%) G3–4: reversible neutropenia (n = 3, 12%), anemia (n = 2, 8%), thrombocytopenia (n = 2, 8%) G1–2: fatigue (n = 16, 62%), sensory neuropathy (n = 14, 54%), nausea (n = 12, 46%), hyperglycemia (n = 11, 42%), allergy reaction (n = 7, 27%), herpes reactivation (n = 1, 4%)

| Zhang et al,[25] 2017 | Retrospective study | IBD | B IV 1.0 mg/m^2, D (40 mg) on d 1, 4, 8, and 11 of a 21-d cycle for at least 4 consecutive cycles Median number of cycles: 8 | 10 | NA | 80% ORR, 1 (10%) CR, 1 (10%) VGPR, 6 (60%) PR mTTR 1.8 mo after m f/u period of 36 mo, 100% OS & 6 had no disease progression mTTP 39 mo | G3 neutropenia (n = 1), G3 anemia (n = 2), G1–2 thrombocytopenia (G2 n = 1, G1 n = 5), G1–2 neuropathy (n = 6, 60%), G2 infection (n = 2) G1–2 edema (n = 4, 40%) G1–2 gastrointestinal disorders |
| Treon et al,[26] 2009 | Phase 2 study | BDR | B: 1.3 mg/m^2 IV, D 40 mg po on d 1, 4, 8, 11, every 21 d, R 375 mg/m^2 on d 11 4 cycles induction & 4 cycles maintenance treatment | 23 | NA | 22 (96%) ORR, 19 (83%) MRR, 3 (13%) CR, 2 (9%) nCR, 3 (13%) VGPR, 11 (48%) PR, 3 (13%) MR mTTP: NR estimated mTTP >30 mo mTTR:1.4 mo m f/u of 22.8 mo, PFS 78.3%, OS 100% | G4 neutropenia (n = 1, 4%), G2 infections without neutropenia (n = 10, 43%), G2–3 peripheral neuropathy (n = 16, 69%), herpes zoster reactivation (n = 5, 22%), G2–3 thrombocytopenia (n = 10, 44%), G2 anemia (n = 18, 78%) |

(continued on next page)

Table 1
(continued)

Study	Type of Study	Regimen	Dose and Schedule of PI	No of Untreated pts	Mutation	Results	Adverse Events of PI
Dimopoulos et al,[28] 2013	Prospective phase 2 multicenter trial	BDR	B 1.3 mg/m² IV on d 1, 4, 8, 11 followed by weekly B 1.6 mg/m² IV on d 1, 8, 15, & 22 every 35 d for 4 cycles, followed by D 40 mg & R IV 375 mg/m² on d 1, 8, 15, & 22 in cycle 2 & 5	59	NA	85% ORR, 68% MRR, 2 (3%) CR, 4 (7%) VGPR, 38 (65%) PR, 10 (17%) MR, 3 (5%) SD, 6 (10%) PD Median time to first response (>MR): 3 mo, median time to best response: 5 mo, 4 (8%) best response 6 mo after completion of therapy m f/u: 42 mo, estimated mPFS:42 mo, 3 y OS: 81%	>G3: neutropenia (15%), sensory neuropathy (7%), infections (7%), respiratory symptoms (10%) 46% fatigue, gastrointestinal disorders
Khwaja et al,[30] 2022	Retrospective multicenter study	BDR, VCD ± R	B (15/27)[a] pts: 1.3 mg/ m², (12/27)[a] pts: 1.6 mg/m² weekly for 3–4 doses per cycle for up to 10 cycles & monthly thereafter Median of 6 cycles	11 BDR 1 VCD ± R	7/8 (88%) MYD88[L265P] 2/3 (67%) CXCR4	92% ORR, 83% MRR, 8% CR, 33% VGPR, 42% PR, 8% MR, 8% SD 2 y OS: 100%, 2 y PFS: 88%	G1–2 neuropathy (n = 3, 25%) G1–2 gastrointestinal disorders (n = 1, 8%)
Castillo et al,[31] 2018	Retrospective comparative study (CDR-BDR-Benda-R)	BDR	BDR: B 1.6 mg/m² IV or SC, D 20 mg IV or po on days 1, 4, 8 d 11, or 1, 8, 15, & 22, every 3 & 4 wk, R 375 mg/m² IV on d 11 or 22, for 4 cycles Maintenance: R	87 BDR	23 (88%) MYD88[L265P] 11 (42%) CXCR4	BDR: 9 (11%) CR, 20 (24%) VGPR, 40 (48%) PR, 6 (7%) MR, 8 (10%) NR Received maintenance: 55 (65%) The median times to best response: 20 mo mPFS 5.8 y, m f/u time: 4 y, m OS: NR	Neuropathy

Abeykoon et al,[7] 2021	Comparative study (Benda-R)-(DRC)-(BDR)	BDR	BDR, 6 cycles (cycle 1: 21 d, cycles 2–5: 35 d per cycle) B 1.3 mg/m² IV or (SC) on d 1, 4, 8, and 11 of cycle 1, & at 1.6 mg/m² in subsequent cycles, D 40 mg on d 1, 8, 15, 22 of the 2 cycle and beyond, R 375 mg/m² IV on d 1, 8, 15, 22 on 2 & 5 cycle	45 BDR	14/24 (58%) $MYD88^{L265P}$	84% ORR, 68% MRR mTTNT 2.6 y, event-free survival: 1.6 y, time to best response: 6.7 mo, estimated mPFS: 1.8 y m f/u for 5.2 y, DOR 3.6 y, 4-y OS 87%	>G3 neuropathy (10.5%), neutropenia (2.5%), fatigue (2.5%), <G3 anemia (2.5%)
Auer et al,[32] 2016	Prospective randomized multicenter, noncomparative phase 2 (BCR-FCR)	BCR	BCR: B 1.6 mg/m² SC days 1, 8, 15, C 250 mg/m² po d 1, 8, 15, R 375 mg/m² IV d 1, 8, 15, 22, cycles 2 and 5 only	42 BCR	NA	97.6% ORR 78.6% MRR CR = 1, VGPR = 8, PR = 24, MR = 7, SD = 1 3 progressed, 1 death	No >G3 neuropathy >G3: anemia (n = 5, 11.9%), neutropenia (n = 11, 26.2%), thrombocytopenia (n = 7, 16.7%), infection (n = 2, 4.8%)
Leblebjian et al,[33] 2015	Retrospective study	CyBorD ± R	Bortezomib: 9/15[a] pts: 1.3 mg/m² on a twice-weekly, 6/15[a] pts weekly on d 1, 8, & 15	4/15 (27%)	NA	1 CR, 1 PR, 2 MR 100% ORR mTTP 18.6 mo	Neuropathy
Buske,[34] 2020	Prospective randomized multicenter European phase 2 study (B-DRC-DRC)	B-DRC	DRC (D 20 mg po d 1, R 375 mg/m² IV d 1 cycle 1 & 1400 mg SC d 1 cycle 2–6, C 100 mg/m² × 2 po d 1–5) & B SC 1,6 mg/m² d 1, 8, 15) for 6 cycles (28 d interval)	101	26/72 $MYD88^{MT}$ & $CXCR4^{WT}$ 8/72 $MYD88^{MT}/CXCR4^{WT}$ 5/72 $MYD88^{WT}/CXCR4^{WT}$	91.2% ORR, 79.1% MRR, 18.7% CR/VGPR mPFS NR, estimated 2-y PFS 80.6%, mOS NR, 5 deaths	G ≥ 3 cytopenia, infection G3 (n = 2) & G1–2 (n = 16) peripheral sensory neuropathy

Abbreviations: B, bortezomib; B-DRC, bortezomib-dexamethasone-rituximab-cyclophosphamide; CyBorD, cyclophosphamide-bortezomib-dexamethasone; D, dexamethasone; G, grade; IBD, low-dose bortezomib-dexamethasone; m f/u, median follow-up; mDOR, median duration of response; mOS, median overall survival; mPFS, median progression-free survival; MT, mutation; mTTNT, median time to next therapy; NA, not available; nCR, near-complete response; NR, not reached; po, per os; pts, patients; R, rituximab; Benda-R, bendamustine-rituximab; SD, stable disease; WT, wild type.
[a] For both untreated/previously treated pts.

follow-up time of 8.5 years, the mTTP was 5.5 years,[27] with a 5-year progression-free survival (PFS) of 57% and 5-year overall survival (OS) of 95%. With the longer follow-up, peripheral neuropathy resolved in 8 out of 16 patients (50%) or improved to G1 in 5 patients.[27]

In a larger phase 2 prospective study, 59 untreated patients received BDR.[28] Unlike the Treon study,[26] maintenance therapy was not given; there was an induction with bortezomib before the addition of rituximab to avoid an IgM flare, and the drug was used weekly at a dose of 1.6 mg/m^2, as an IV infusion. The ORR was 85%, and a major response was attained in 68% of patients. Sensory neuropathy developed in almost half of the patients (46%), with 4 (7%) having neuropathy grade 3 or higher. Other common adverse events included fatigue and gastrointestinal disorders. After administering rituximab in the second cycle, a $\geq$25% elevation of IgM was recorded in 11% of the enrolled patients, with the median absolute increase being 1614 mg/dL; however, none of the patients needed to undergo plasmapheresis. This was attributed to the initial induction with bortezomib, which reduced IgM levels by a median of 18%, allowing a safer introduction of rituximab in cycle 2. The final results of this study, after a median follow-up of 86 months, showed a median PFS of 43 months, but the DOR in patients who achieved at least PR was 64.5 months and the OS rate at 7 years was 66%.[29] The sensory neuropathy resolved or decreased to grade 1 in all patients. Moreover, disease transformation to diffuse large B-cell lymphoma was recorded in 3 patients, but none developed secondary myelodysplasia. In a retrospective study,[30] 11 patients received BDR, and one patient received bortezomib, cyclophosphamide, and dexamethasone (VCD) as frontline therapy. ORR and MRR were 92% and 83%, respectively. After 2 years, all patients (100%) were alive, and the 2-year PFS was 88%. Regarding side effects, neuropathy grade 1 to 2 was observed in 3 patients (25%), and one patient (8%) had gastrointestinal disorders grade 1 to 2. Furthermore, secondary myelodysplastic syndrome was not observed.

There are limited studies that prospectively compare regimens with versus without bortezomib and somewhat more data from retrospective studies. A retrospective study by Castillo and colleagues[31] compared the outcomes in patients who received primary therapy with cyclophosphamide, dexamethasone, and rituximab (DRC), BDR, and bendamustine and rituximab (Benda-R). Among 87 patients treated with BDR, 11% achieved complete response (CR), 24% achieved very good partial response (VGPR), and 48% achieved partial response (PR). The median PFS was 5.8 years, and at a median follow-up interval of 4 years, the estimated 5-year OS rate was 96%. Even though 58 patients received bortezomib twice a week and 29 patients received bortezomib once per week, there was no difference in the response rates and PFS between them. Neuropathy was the most common toxicity, which improved in frequency by modification of the dose or the route of administration of bortezomib. Compared with the other treatment combinations (BR and DRC), there was no difference in the response rates. However, the patients on BDR and Benda-R attained the best response faster. Patients that received Benda-R had numerically longer median PFS than those treated with BDR and DRC (5.8, 5.5, and 4.8 years, respectively). However, between BDR and DRC, the difference was not statistically significant (log-rank P = .69).[31] Abeykoon and colleagues[7] compared data from treatment-naïve patients that received Benda-R, BDR, or DRC. In the BDR group, *MYD88* mutations were linked to better ORR (75% in *MYD88*^{L256P} vs 67% in *MYD88*^{WT}). The data revealed that the Benda-R regimen compared with BDR and DRC was superior in terms of MRR (96%, 68%, 53%, respectively), time to best response, and PFS (median, 5.2, 1.8, 4.3 years, respectively). The EFS was not reached in the Benda-R group, whereas the BDR and DRC groups were 1.6 and 4.3 years. Time to next therapy (TTNT) and DOR were not reached in patients with Benda-R; in the BDR group, these parameters were 2.6 and 3.6 years, respectively, and in the DRC group were 4.4 and 3.9 years, respectively. Moreover, bortezomib was discontinued in 2 patients owing to neurotoxicity.

In another study, Auer and colleagues[32] found that treatment-naïve patients who were administered SC bortezomib in combination with cyclophosphamide and rituximab (BCR) achieved high response rates (98% ORR and 79% MRR). This prospective, randomized study revealed that the efficacy of BCR seemed similar to the combination of fludarabine, cyclophosphamide, and rituximab (FCR) with 82.4% of patients reaching ORR and 76.5% of patients reaching MRR. The BCR regimen was not associated with grade 3 neuropathy.[32] Notably, myelodysplastic syndrome occurred in 2 patients treated with FCR, leading to their deaths. A retrospective study by Leblebjian and colleagues[33] evaluated bortezomib in combination with cyclophosphamide and dexamethasone (n = 15). In 7 patients, rituximab was added. Among 4 previously untreated patients with WM, one achieved CR, one achieved PR, and 2 achieved minor responses (MRs), with ORR reaching 100%. The mTTP was 18.6 months, and the most common toxicity was neuropathy.[33]

The European Consortium for WM[34] conducted a prospective randomized clinical trial comparing DRC with DRC plus bortezomib SC. DRC remains a standard therapeutic regimen for previously untreated patients with WM, and in this study, was given every 4 weeks (instead of every 3 weeks in the original publication). In the experimental arm, bortezomib was given SC at a dose of 1.6 mg/m^2 on days 1, 8, and 15 for 6 cycles in addition to DRC. In cycle 1, rituximab 375 mg/m^2 was administered IV on day 1 and in the subsequent cycles 2 to 6 at a dose of 1400 mg SC on day 1. The study enrolled 202 patients (101 in DRC and 101 in B-DRC arm). The results showed that ORR and MRR were attained in 91% and 79% of patients treated with B-DRC, whereas the response rates in the DRC group were 86.7% and 68.9%, respectively. PFS was not reached in patients with B-DRC regimen, whereas PFS in DRC was 50.1 months, with the estimated PFS at 24 months being comparable at 81% and 73%, respectively. The mutation status of the *MYD88* and *CXCR4* genes impacted neither the response rates nor the PFS. Both regimens were well-tolerated. Among patients who received B-DRC, 43% experienced grade 3 or higher adverse events. Sensory neuropathy grade 3 occurred in 2 patients, whereas sensory neuropathy grade 1 to 2 occurred in 16 patients.

Carfilzomib

Carfilzomib is a second-generation tetrapeptide epoxyketone PI that, unlike bortezomib, irreversibly inhibits the 20S proteasome subunit.[35] It is administered IV and is a neuropathy-sparing option. However, cardiotoxicity has been described in 3% to 4% of patients with MM treated with carfilzomib, and thrombotic microangiopathy has been observed in several studies. Hence, attention should be paid to elderly patients with preexisting cardiovascular disease.[36,37] Carfilzomib has been approved by the Food and Drug Administration (FDA) for MM as a single agent or in combination with dexamethasone or dexamethasone and lenalidomide.

Treon and colleagues[38] investigated carfilzomib in combination with rituximab and dexamethasone (CaRD) in a prospective study (**Table 2**). Carfilzomib was given in 3-week cycles on days 1, 2, 8, and 9 for 8 induction cycles, followed by maintenance treatment on days 1 and 2 every 8 weeks for 8 cycles. Thirty-one patients were enrolled, and 28 patients were previously untreated. ORR and MRR were 89% and 71%, respectively, and were not influenced by *MYD88*[L256P] or *CXCR4*[WHIM] mutation status. At a median follow-up time of 15.4 months, no patient had died. The most

Table 2
Clinical studies of carfilzomib in previously untreated patients with Waldenström macroglobulinemia

Study	Type of Study	Regimen	Dose and Schedule of PI	No. of Untreated pts.	Mutation	Results	Adverse Events of PI
Treon et.al.[38] 2014	Prospective, open-label, single stage, phase 2 study	CaRD	Ca IV 20 mg/m² (cycle 1) & 36 mg/m² (cycles 2–6), D IV 20 mg, on d 1, 2, 8, & 9, R 375 mg/m², on d 2 & 9 every 21 d Maintenance therapy: IV Ca 36 mg/m², IV D 20 mg, on d 1 & 2, R 375 mg/m², on d 2 every 8 wk for 8 cycles	28/31 (90.3%)	29/30 (96.6%)[a] MYD88^L265P 11/30 (36.7%)[a] CXCR4^WHIM	25/28 (89.2%) ORR, 20/28 (71.4%) MRR, 1/28 (3.5%) CR, 9/28 (32.1%) VGPR, 9/28 (32.1%) PR, 6/28 (21.4%) MR m f/u of 15.4 mo: no deaths, OS 100%	G1-3 hyperlipasemia, hyperamylasemia neutropenia G3 cardiomyopathy[a] G2 hyperbilirubinemia
Chaudhry et al,[40] 2019	Retrospective, single-center study	CaRD	Ca IV 20 mg/m² (cycle 1) & 36 mg/m² (cycles 2–6), D IV 20 mg, on d 1, 2, 8, & 9, R 375 mg/m², on d 2 & 9 every 21 d Maintenance therapy: IV Ca 36 mg/m², IV D 20 mg, on d 1 & 2, R 375 mg/m², on d 2 every 8 wk for 8 cycles	6	5/6 (83%) MYD88 0 CXCR4	67% MRR, 1 (17%) CR, 3 (50%) PR, 2 (33%) MR At an m f/u of 33.5 mo: OS 100% & PFS 66%	No neuropathy & cardiomyopathy

Abbreviation: Ca, carfilzomib.
[a] For both untreated/previously treated pts.

common adverse effects were asymptomatic hyperlipasemia, often accompanied with elevated amylase, neutropenia, possibly attributed to carfilzomib, and one patient developed cardiomyopathy. Hyperlipasemia and hyperamylasemia led to the reduction of the dose of carfilzomib in affected patients. Only neuropathy grade 1 and 2 was recorded, and no patient required discontinuation of the treatment because of neuropathy, suggesting that carfilzomib is associated with a low risk for neurotoxicity, in contrast to bortezomib.[38] Long-term results[39] from the study confirmed similarly high response rates; the median PFS was achieved at 46 months, and all patients were still alive. There were no additional safety concerns, suggesting that carfilzomib could be an active, well-tolerated, and neuropathy-sparing treatment option. However, cardiac toxicity should always be considered.[39]

In the prospective study of Chaudhry and colleagues,[40] six untreated patients with symptomatic WM received the combination CaRD. Even though 80% were positive for $MYD88^{L265P}$ mutation, the researchers claimed that the mutational status did not influence the treatment's response. Of patients, 67% achieved MRR, and all had a clinical benefit as anemia and B symptoms resolved. At a median follow-up of 34 months, all patients were alive, and PFS was 66%. No cardiomyopathy was noted. Hence, the researchers suggested that carfilzomib could be a good first-line treatment choice because it led to high response rates, and it seemed to be well-tolerated.[40]

Ixazomib

Ixazomib is an orally administered boronic acid analogue of bortezomib that reversibly binds to the β5 subunit of the 20S proteasome. It received approval from the the FDA for treating relapsed or refractory MM in combination with lenalidomide and dexamethasone. The clinical results of ixazomib as a first-line therapy in WM are described in **Table 3**.

Castillo and colleagues,[41] in a prospective phase 2 study, administered ixazomib in combination with dexamethasone and rituximab (IDR) in 26 symptomatic, previously untreated WM patients. Ixazomib was given orally at a dose of 4 mg on days 1, 8, and 15 every 4 weeks for 6 cycles as induction therapy, followed by 6 cycles every 8 weeks as maintenance therapy. Rituximab therapy started after 2 cycles of ixazomib and dexamethasone to reduce the risk of an IgM flare. All patients harbored $MYD88^{L265P}$ mutation, whereas 15 (58%) patients carried $CXCR4$ mutations. The ORR was 96% (including 15% VGPR, 62% PR, and 19% MR); the depth of response was related to PFS duration. No grade 4 adverse effects were reported, and most of the adverse events were grade 1 to 2 infusion reactions attributed to rituximab in 39% of patients and nausea in 35% of patients. The long-term results of this study showed that VGPR and PR rates improved to 19% and 58%, respectively.[42] After a median follow-up of 52 months, median PFS, DOR, and TTNT were 40, 38, and 40 months and were not influenced by the $CXCR4$ mutations. Ixazomib was not associated with neuropathy or adverse cardiovascular events in this study, and no grade 4 toxicities or deaths were recorded. Hence, the researchers suggested that the IDR combination is a safe, well-tolerated, and effective option for treatment-naïve patients with WM. Alloo and colleagues[43] presented 2 cases, one patient with MM and another with WM, who developed cutaneous necrotizing vasculitis with ixazomib use, that resolved after a reduction in the dose of ixazomib.

NEW PROTEASOME INHIBITORS

Oprozomib is an oral tripeptide epoxyketone PI, analogous to carfilzomib. It binds irreversibly to the proteasome and activates caspases 3, 8, and 9 and poly(ADP) ribose

Table 3
Clinical studies of ixazomib in previously untreated patients with Waldenström macroglobulinemia

Study	Type of Study	Regimen	Dose and Schedule of PI	No. of Untreated pts.	Mutation	Results	Adverse Events of PI
Castillo et al,[41] 2018	Prospective investigator-initiated phase 2 study	IDR	po I 4 mg + IV or po D 20 mg on d 1, 8, & 15 every 4 wk for induction cycles 1 and 2 + IV R 375 mg/m^2 on d 1, every 4 wk for cycles 3–6 Maintenance therapy: every 8 wk for 6 cycles	26 symptomatic	26 (100%) MYD88^{L265P} 15 (58%) CXCR4	25 (96%) ORR, 20 (77%) MRR, 0 CR, 4 (15%) VGPR, 62% PR, 19% MR, 7 PD mTTR: 8 wk, mPFS: NR at m f/u of 22 mo	No G4 G3: neuropathy (n = 1, 3%), pneumonia (n = 1, 3%), sepsis (n = 1, 3%) G1 & 2: infusion reactions (n = 10, 38.5%), nausea (n = 9, 34.6%), insomnia (n = 7, 26.9%), rash (n = 7, 26.9%)

Abbreviations: I, ixazomib; PD, progressive disease.

polymerase and prevents the chymotrypsin-like activity of the proteasome, migration, and angiogenesis.[44] Moreover, oprozomib seems to have bone-anabolic activity and reduces bone resorption.[45] Oprozomib has not been studied in previously untreated patients with WM, and the experience is limited in the relapsed setting, especially owing to an increased risk of gastrointestinal adverse events, which included 3 events of death associated with gastrointestinal hemorrhage deemed to be related to oprozomib.[46] Oprozomib is no longer being developed for the treatment of plasma cell dyscrasias.

Marizomib is a beta-lactone, irreversible PI.[47] Marizomib has yet shown activity only in preclinical settings. Roccaro and colleagues[48] showed that marizomib induced cytotoxicity in patients' WM cells and did not harm the normal peripheral blood mononuclear cells. The cytotoxicity was triggered by dose-dependent apoptosis through caspase-8 and PARP cleavage without acting on caspases-3 and -9. In addition, marizomib downregulated the antiapoptotic protein Mcl-1 and increased the second mitochondria-derived activator of caspases (Smac/DIABLO) from mitochondria to cytosol. However, clinical data on marizomib in WM are lacking.

SUMMARY

PIs have now been used for almost 20 years in the treatment of myeloma and other plasma cell dyscrasias as well as in the treatment of WM. Their use has been associated with a significant improvement in the survival of patients with MM, and PIs are part of backbone therapies in every disease setting. In WM, PIs are not a backbone therapy, although their use is associated with certain benefits. PI-containing regimens rapidly decrease IgM levels, reduce the risk of IgM flare, and do not expose patients to the risk of significant short- or long-term myelotoxicity, thus providing a "chemotherapy-free" option. On the other hand, administration of bortezomib is associated with a significant risk of neurotoxicity and carfilzomib with a risk of cardiac toxicity, while both drugs require weekly administration (depending on the setting, in a hospital environment) for a fixed, yet long, duration of therapy. Ixazomib is a new option with convenience in terms of administration (given weekly orally), but still with some gastrointestinal toxicity. The pros and cons of these agents should be viewed also in the context of the available treatment options for WM, which include chemoimmunotherapy and BTKis, as well as upcoming BCL2 inhibitors. Bortezomib combinations with rituximab offer a fixed duration, low-cost, chemotherapy-free alternative regimen for selected patients, which is probably noninferior to DRC. With appropriate measures (weekly administration and close follow-up for neuropathy), this regimen can be considered for patients with cytopenias, cardiovascular diseases, WM-related amyloidosis, or other IgM-related complications. The results of the ECWM-1 showed that the added benefit of bortezomib to an effective chemoimmunotherapy regimen, such as DRC, is not substantial. Still, the combination may have a role in managing some patient subgroups without significantly increasing toxicity. Patients with AL amyloidosis, cryoglobulinemia, cold agglutinin disease, and those presenting with high IgM levels who may not be optimal candidates for BTKis or Benda-R owing to concurrent cardiovascular issues and myelotoxicity, respectively, may be candidates for bortezomib-containing therapy. Ixazomib may offer a more convenient but significantly more expensive option than bortezomib. Given its weekly IV administration and cardiac toxicity risk, carfilzomib is not attractive. Given the central role of BTKis and chemoimmunotherapies today, the role of PI-based combinations as primary therapy for WM may be less critical. However, combinations of BTKis with PIs are being explored in prospective clinical trials (NCT04263480). Based on preclinical data, such combinations could induce deep hematologic responses, which cannot be achieved by BKTis alone, and perhaps offer an opportunity for a fixed duration regimen or at least allow safer discontinuation of BTKis. The impact of genotype (*MYD88* and *CXCR4* mutations) should also be investigated further to elucidate if these mutations play a role in the efficacy of PIs, and current data on this topic are limited.

In conclusion, although the treatment approach for WM is changing, PIs remain a treatment option for select patients with WM. In an individualized therapy approach, PIs can be a part of chemotherapy-containing or chemotherapy-free, fixed-duration regimens for patients not eligible for chemotherapy or at high risk for IgM-related complications.

CLINICS CARE POINTS

- The use of PIs in WM is associated with certain benefits since they rapidly decrease IgM levels, reduce the risk of IgM flare and are considered as a chemotherapy-free treatment option.
- Bortezomib is associated with neurotoxicity, while carfilzomib with cardiac toxicity.
- Ixazomib is given weekly orally and its gastrointestinal toxicity should be taken into consideration.
- The use of PIs should be viewed in the context of the available treatment options and the choice of each regimen should be individualized.

REFERENCES

1. Kasi PM, Ansell SM, Gertz MA. Waldenström macroglobulinemia. Clin Adv Hematol Oncol 2015;13(1):56–66.
2. Owen RG, Treon SP, Al-Katib A, et al. Clinicopathological definition of Waldenstrom's macroglobulinemia: Consensus Panel Recommendations from the Second International Workshop on Waldenstrom's Macroglobulinemia. Semin Oncol 2003;30(2):110–5.
3. Castillo JJ, Olszewski AJ, Kanan S, et al. Overall survival and competing risks of death in patients with Waldenström macroglobulinaemia: an analysis of the Surveillance, Epidemiology and End Results database. Br J Haematol 2015;169(1):81–9.
4. Simon L, Baron M, Leblond V. How we manage patients with Waldenström macroglobulinaemia. Br J Haematol 2018;181(6):737–51.
5. Gertz MA. Waldenström macroglobulinemia. Hematol Amst Neth 2012;17(Suppl 1):S112–6.
6. Castillo JJ, Treon SP. What is new in the treatment of Waldenstrom macroglobulinemia? Leukemia 2019;33(11):2555–62.
7. Abeykoon JP, Zanwar S, Ansell SM, et al. Assessment of fixed-duration therapies for treatment-naïve Waldenström macroglobulinemia. Am J Hematol 2021;96(8):945–53.
8. Kastritis E, Gavriatopoulou M, Kyrtsonis MC, et al. Dexamethasone, rituximab, and cyclophosphamide as primary treatment of Waldenström macroglobulinemia: final analysis of a phase 2 study. Blood 2015;126(11):1392–4.
9. Rummel MJ, Al-Batran SE, Kim SZ, et al. Bendamustine plus rituximab is effective and has a favorable toxicity profile in the treatment of mantle cell and low-grade non-Hodgkin's lymphoma. J Clin Oncol 2005;23(15):3383–9.

10. Treon SP, Tripsas CK, Meid K, et al. Ibrutinib in previously treated Waldenström's macroglobulinemia. N Engl J Med 2015;372(15):1430–40.

11. Leleu X, Eeckhoute J, Jia X, et al. Targeting NF-kappaB in Waldenstrom macroglobulinemia. Blood 2008;111(10):5068–77.

12. Mitsiades CS, Mitsiades N, Hideshima T, et al. Proteasome inhibition as a therapeutic strategy for hematologic malignancies. Expert Rev Anticancer Ther 2005; 5(3):465–76.

13. Adams J. The development of proteasome inhibitors as anticancer drugs. Cancer Cell 2004;5(5):417–21.

14. Kuhn DJ, Chen Q, Voorhees PM, et al. Potent activity of carfilzomib, a novel, irreversible inhibitor of the ubiquitin-proteasome pathway, against preclinical models of multiple myeloma. Blood 2007;110(9):3281–90.

15. Mitsiades N, Mitsiades CS, Richardson PG, et al. The proteasome inhibitor PS-341 potentiates sensitivity of multiple myeloma cells to conventional chemotherapeutic agents: therapeutic applications. Blood 2003;101(6):2377–80.

16. Rajkumar SV, Richardson PG, Hideshima T, et al. Proteasome inhibition as a novel therapeutic target in human cancer. J Clin Oncol 2005;23(3):630–9.

17. Lee AH, Iwakoshi NN, Anderson KC, et al. Proteasome inhibitors disrupt the unfolded protein response in myeloma cells. Proc Natl Acad Sci U S A 2003; 100(17):9946–51.

18. Meister S, Schubert U, Neubert K, et al. Extensive immunoglobulin production sensitizes myeloma cells for proteasome inhibition. Cancer Res 2007;67(4): 1783–92.

19. Nakagawa T, Zhu H, Morishima N, et al. Caspase-12 mediates endoplasmic-reticulum-specific apoptosis and cytotoxicity by amyloid-beta. Nature 2000; 403(6765):98–103.

20. Pham LV, Tamayo AT, Yoshimura LC, et al. Inhibition of constitutive NF-kappa B activation in mantle cell lymphoma B cells leads to induction of cell cycle arrest and apoptosis. J Immunol Baltim Md 1950 2003;171(1):88–95.

21. Chen CI, Kouroukis CT, White D, et al. Bortezomib is active in patients with untreated or relapsed Waldenstrom's macroglobulinemia: a phase II study of the National Cancer Institute of Canada Clinical Trials Group. J Clin Oncol 2007; 25(12):1570–5.

22. Treon SP, Hunter ZR, Matous J, et al. Multicenter clinical trial of bortezomib in relapsed/refractory Waldenstrom's macroglobulinemia: results of WMCTG Trial 03-248. Clin Cancer Res 2007;13(11):3320–5.

23. Ghobrial IM, Xie W, Padmanabhan S, et al. Phase II trial of weekly bortezomib in combination with rituximab in untreated patients with Waldenström Macroglobulinemia. Am J Hematol 2010;85(9):670–4.

24. CTG Labs - NCBI. Available at: https://beta.clinicaltrials.gov/study/NCT004227 99?tab=results. Accessed January 23, 2023.

25. Zhang YP, Yang X, Lin ZH, et al. Low-dose bortezomib and dexamethasone as primary therapy in elderly patients with Waldenström macroglobulinemia. Eur J Haematol 2017;99(6):489–94.

26. Treon SP, Ioakimidis L, Soumerai JD, et al. Primary therapy of Waldenström macroglobulinemia with bortezomib, dexamethasone, and rituximab: WMCTG clinical trial 05-180. J Clin Oncol 2009;27(23):3830–5.

27. Treon SP. Long-Term Outcome of a Prospective Study of Bortezomib, Dexamethasone and Rituximab (BDR) in Previously Untreated, Symptomatic Patients with Waldenstrom's Macroglobulinemia. Published 2015. Available at: https://ash.confex.

com/ash/2015/webprogramscheduler/Paper86155.html. Accessed November 6, 2022.

28. Dimopoulos MA, García-Sanz R, Gavriatopoulou M, et al. Primary therapy of Waldenstrom macroglobulinemia (WM) with weekly bortezomib, low-dose dexamethasone, and rituximab (BDR): long-term results of a phase 2 study of the European Myeloma Network (EMN). Blood 2013;122(19):3276–82.

29. Gavriatopoulou M, García-Sanz R, Kastritis E, et al. BDR in newly diagnosed patients with WM: final analysis of a phase 2 study after a minimum follow-up of 6 years. Blood 2017;129(4):456–9.

30. Khwaja J, Uppal E, Baker R, et al. Bortezomib-based therapy is effective and well tolerated in frontline and multiply pre-treated Waldenström macroglobulinaemia including BTKi failures: A real-world analysis - Khwaja - 2022 - eJHaem - Wiley Online Library. Available at: https://onlinelibrary.wiley.com/doi/full/10.1002/jha2.597. Accessed January 23, 2023.

31. Castillo JJ, Gustine JN, Meid K, et al. Response and survival for primary therapy combination regimens and maintenance rituximab in Waldenström macroglobulinaemia. Br J Haematol 2018;181(1):77–85.

32. Auer RL, Owen RG, D'Sa S, et al. R2W: Subcutaneous Bortezomib, Cyclophosphamide and Rituximab (BCR) Versus Fludarabine, Cyclophosphamide and Rituximab (FCR) for Initial Therapy of Waldenstrőm's Macroglobulinemia: A Randomised Phase II Study. Blood 2016;128(22):618.

33. Leblebjian H, Noonan K, Paba-Prada C, et al. Cyclophosphamide, bortezomib, and dexamethasone combination in Waldenstrom macroglobulinemia. Am J Hematol 2015;90(6):E122–3.

34. Christian Buske. Bortezomib in Combination with Dexamethasone, Rituximab and Cyclophosphamide (B-DRC) As First - Line Treatment of Waldenstrom's Macroglobulinemia: Results of a Prospectively Randomized Multicenter European Phase II Trial | Blood | American Society of Hematology. Published 2020. Available at: https://ashpublications.org/blood/article/136/Supplement%201/26/469992/Bortezomib-in-Combination-with-Dexamethasone. Accessed November 13, 2022.

35. Gavriatopoulou M, Terpos E, Kastritis E, et al. Current treatment options and investigational drugs for Waldenstrom's Macroglobulinemia. Expert Opin Investig Drugs 2017;26(2):197–205.

36. Castillo JJ, Advani RH, Branagan AR, et al. Consensus treatment recommendations from the tenth International Workshop for Waldenström Macroglobulinaemia. Lancet Haematol 2020;7(11):e827–37.

37. Leblond V, Kastritis E, Advani R, et al. Treatment recommendations from the Eighth International Workshop on Waldenström's Macroglobulinemia. Blood 2016;128(10):1321–8.

38. Treon SP, Tripsas CK, Meid K, et al. Carfilzomib, rituximab, and dexamethasone (CaRD) treatment offers a neuropathy-sparing approach for treating Waldenström's macroglobulinemia. Blood 2014;124(4):503–10.

39. Meid. Long-Term Follow-up of a Prospective Clinical Trial of Carfilzomib, Rituximab and Dexamethasone (CaRD) in Waldenstrom's Macroglobulinemia | Blood | American Society of Hematology. Published 2017. Available at: https://ashpublications.org/blood/article/130/Supplement%201/2772/80469/Long-Term-Follow-up-of-a-Prospective-Clinical. Accessed November 6, 2022.

40. Chaudhry M, Steiner R, Claussen C, et al. Carfilzomib-based combination regimens are highly effective frontline therapies for multiple myeloma and Waldenström's macroglobulinemia. Leuk Lymphoma 2019;60(4):964–70.

41. Castillo JJ, Meid K, Gustine JN, et al. Prospective Clinical Trial of Ixazomib, Dexamethasone, and Rituximab as Primary Therapy in Waldenström Macroglobulinemia. Clin Cancer Res 2018;24(14):3247–52.
42. Castillo JJ, Meid K, Flynn CA, et al. Ixazomib, dexamethasone, and rituximab in treatment-naive patients with Waldenström macroglobulinemia: long-term follow-up. Blood Adv 2020;4(16):3952–9.
43. Alloo A, Khosravi H, Granter SR, et al. Ixazomib-induced cutaneous necrotizing vasculitis. Support Care Cancer 2018;26(7):2247–50.
44. Chauhan D, Singh AV, Aujay M, et al. A novel orally active proteasome inhibitor ONX 0912 triggers in vitro and in vivo cytotoxicity in multiple myeloma. Blood 2010;116(23):4906–15.
45. Hurchla MA, Garcia-Gomez A, Hornick MC, et al. The epoxyketone-based proteasome inhibitors carfilzomib and orally bioavailable oprozomib have anti-resorptive and bone-anabolic activity in addition to anti-myeloma effects. Leukemia 2013;27(2):430–40.
46. Ghobrial IM, Vij R, Siegel D, et al. A Phase Ib/II Study of Oprozomib in Patients with Advanced Multiple Myeloma and Waldenström Macroglobulinemia. Clin Cancer Res 2019;25(16):4907–16.
47. Boccadoro M. Second-generation Proteasome Inhibition: What a Difference a Generation Makes. Clin Lymphoma Myeloma. Leuk 2015;15:e13–4. https://doi.org/10.1016/j.clml.2015.08.029.
48. Roccaro AM, Leleu X, Sacco A, et al. Dual targeting of the proteasome regulates survival and homing in Waldenstrom macroglobulinemia. Blood 2008;111(9):4752–63.

BTK Inhibitors in the Frontline Management of Waldenström Macroglobulinemia

Marzia Varettoni, MD[a],*, Jeffrey V. Matous, MD[b]

KEYWORDS

- Waldenström macroglobulinemia • Untreated • Frontline therapy • BTK inhibitors
- Ibrutinib • Acalabrutinib • Zanubrutinib • Tirabrutinib

KEY POINTS

- Bruton Kinase (BTK) inhibitors have demonstrated clinically meaningful efficacy in patients with previously untreated Waldenström macroglobulinemia.
- Compared with ibrutinib, zanubrutinib provided faster and deeper response in patients with CXCR4 mutations.
- Second-generation BTK inhibitors, acalabrutinib and zanubrutinib, have also shown activity in MYD88 Wild type (WT) patients.
- Safety profile of acalabrutinib and zanubrutinib is superior compared with ibrutinib, consistent with lesser off-target activity.

INTRODUCTION

The seminal discovery of the importance of BTK signaling through MYD88 in the pathogenesis of Waldenström macroglobulinemia (WM) ushered in a new era in the treatment of this rare non-Hodgkin lymphoma. Treon and others in 2012 described a recurring, activating somatic mutation in the MYD88 gene, L265P, present in more than 90% of patients with WM, demonstrating its importance in the proliferation and survival of the malignant clone.[1] In their article reporting this discovery, the authors noted, "It remains to be seen whether MYD88 L265P signaling can be targeted for the therapy of Waldenström's macroglobulinemia and non-IgM LPL." It did not take long.

A first-in-class BTK inhibitor (BTKi), ibrutinib, demonstrated remarkable efficacy in previously treated WM as reported by Treon colleagues in 63 patients in 2015,[2] which resulted in approval by the FDA that same year and by European Medicines Agency (EMA) in 2016. By then, whole genome sequencing had uncovered a second mutated

[a] Division of Hematology, Fondazione IRCCS Policlinico San Matteo, Via Golgi 19, 27100 Pavia, Italy; [b] Colorado Blood Cancer Institute, Sarah Cannon Research Institute, Denver, CO, USA
* Corresponding author.
E-mail address: m.varettoni@smatteo.pv.it

Hematol Oncol Clin N Am 37 (2023) 707–717
https://doi.org/10.1016/j.hoc.2023.04.005
0889-8588/23/© 2023 Elsevier Inc. All rights reserved.

gene, CXCR4, found in approximately 30% to 40% of patients with WM, the presence of which conferred a different phenotype. Moreover, patients harboring a CXCR4 mutation seemed to have an attenuated response to ibrutinib, with fewer, less robust, and more delayed responses. Treon and colleagues updated the data from their pivotal trial in 2021 and demonstrated the negative impact of CXCR4 mutations on ibrutinib efficacy.[3] The 5-year progression-free survival (PFS) for patients with MYD88 mutations both without and with CXCR4 mutations was 70% versus 38%, respectively. The efficacy of ibrutinib in the treatment of rituximab-refractory patients with WM was furthermore confirmed by arm C of the iNNOVATE study[4] (discussed below and elsewhere) and other subsequent study. Clinical trials utilizing ibrutinib in previously untreated patients with WM shortly followed.[5,6]

This review will address the role of ibrutinib as well as the next-generation inhibitors of BTK acalabrutinib, zanubrutinib, and tirabrutinib in the treatment of treatment-naïve (TN) patients with WM.

CURRENT EVIDENCE WITH BTK INHIBITORS AS INITIAL THERAPY FOR SYMPTOMATIC WALDENSTRÖM MACROGLOBULINEMIA
Ibrutinib

Data regarding ibrutinib therapy in the first line or TN patients with WM emanate primarily from 3 prospective studies, each of which differ in design but from which one can draw important and similar conclusions (**Table 1**).

In 2018, for the first time, data addressing the use of ibrutinib monotherapy in TN patients with WM were reported. Treon and colleagues published their single-center, prospective experience with first-line ibrutinib in 30 patients.[5] All patients met International Workshop for Waldenström Macroglobulinemia (IWWM) criteria for initiating therapy and the median age was 67 years (range: 43–83). All patients harbored the MYD88 L265P mutation. In addition, 14 patients (47%) had a concomitant CXCR4 mutation. The specific CXCR4 mutations were not initially reported. The primary endpoint was major response rate (MRR). Among the key secondary endpoints was the effect of

Table 1
Efficacy of BTK inhibitors in previously untreated patients with Waldenström macroglobulinemia

	N of Pts	Median Follow-Up (months)	ORR (%)	MRR (%)	CR + VGPR Rate (%)	PFS Rate (%)
Ibrutinib monotherapy						
Castillo, Leukemia 2022[6]	30	50.1	100	87	30	76% at 48 mo
Tam, Blood 2020[11,a]	18	19.4	89	67	17	94% at 18 mo
Ibrutinib + Rituximab						
Buske, JCO 2022[9]	34	50	91	76	27	70% at 48 mo
Acalabrutinib						
Owen, Lancet Haematol 2020[18]	14	63.7	93	78	7	84% at 66 mo
Zanubrutinib						
Trotman, Blood 2020[13]	24	23.5	100	87	33	91% at 24 mo
Tam, Blood 2020[11,a]	19	19.4	94	73	26	78% at 18 mo

[a] Updated at ASCO 2022.

CXCR4 mutational status on response. Responses were judged according to IWWM-6 criteria. All subjects received oral ibrutinib 420 mg daily until progression or tolerance dictated otherwise.

In the initial publication from 2018, with a median follow-up of 13.4 months, all patients (100%) responded to ibrutinib monotherapy, 83% attained a major response, whereas 17% demonstrated minor responses. Responses as judged by a reduction in Immunoglobulin M (IgM) levels and improvements in hemoglobin were brisk: the median times to a minor and major ($\geq$ partial response) response in IgM were 1 month and 1.9 months, respectively. CXCR4 mutations adversely affected both the depth of and time to response. Hemoglobin concentrations increased quickly, with marked improvements by cycle 2, regardless of CXCR4 mutational status (**Fig. 1**). No complete responses were noted.

The authors subsequently updated their findings with a longer median follow-up of 50 months.[6] Of the 14 patients with CXCR4 mutations, 13 had nonsense mutations, whereas 1 had a frameshift mutation. Nonsense CXCR4 mutations confer more BTKi resistance than do frameshift mutations.[7] With longer follow-up, no complete responses were reported but the very good partial response (VGPR) rate increased from 20% to 30% and the MRR had increased from 83% to 87%. The PFS rate at 4 years was 76%. Patients lacking CXCR4 mutations fared the best regarding time to response, depth of response, and PFS.

Tolerance of ibrutinib was excellent with 87% of subjects remaining on therapy at a median treatment duration of 13.4 months in the initial report. Dose reductions were uncommon (10%). At the end of the planned 4-year period of study, 66% remained on active treatment before transitioning to commercial ibrutinib. Side effects of interest included atrial fibrillation (increased from 10% in the 2018 report to 20% with longer follow-up) and hypertension (13%). Two patients progressed early on study, both of whom had CXCR4 mutations.

The phase III iNNOVATE study provided more information regarding the role of ibrutinib in TN patients with WM.[8] However, patients were treated with ibrutinib in combination with rituximab. At the time this study was conceived, single agent rituximab was the most common regimen chosen in the United States for the primary therapy for WM. This double-blind, randomized phase III study included TN patients and previously treated patients. In the latter group, those with known rituximab refractory disease received ibrutinib monotherapy (subgroup C); all other patients were randomized between rituximab and placebo or ibrutinib and rituximab (IR). One hundred fifty patients were included in the phase III portion of the study and randomized, 34 (45%) of whom were treatment naïve. Subjects randomized to ibrutinib plus rituximab received ibrutinib 420 mg orally daily and rituximab at 375 mg/m^2 for a total of 8 doses at weeks 1 to 4 and 17 to 20. Subsequently, more mature data with more than 4 years of follow-up were published; the MRR for the TN patients was 76% and the VGPR rate was 24%.[9] One of the 34 patients (3%) attained a complete remission (CR). Again, responses were rapid with the median times to any response and major response of 1 and 3 months, respectively. The 48-month PFS rate was 70%, in the previously untreated patients similar to the PFS rates in the relapsed patients (71% at 4 years). No new safety signals were seen, and the study confirmed previous experience with ibrutinib therapy for WM: 11% of patients discontinued due to an adverse event (AE), 19% developed any grade of atrial fibrillation, 25% any grade hypertension, and the risk of developing side effects appeared to diminish with prolonged ibrutinib administration.

The iNNOVATE trial yielded several provocative findings. From a safety and tolerability perspective, the addition of ibrutinib to rituximab decreased the incidence of

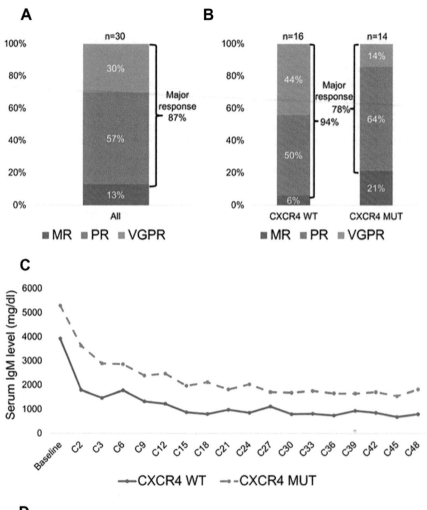

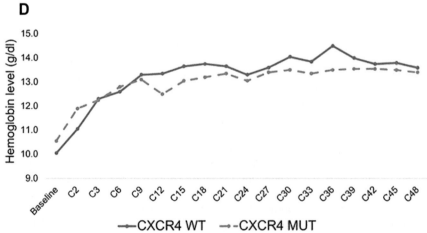

Fig. 1. Response to therapy. Categorical responses at the best response in 30 TN patients with WM treated with ibrutinib for the entire cohort (*A*), by CXCR4 mutational status (*B*), by serial IgM levels (*C*), and hemoglobin levels (*D*). MR, minor response; PR partial response; VGPR, very good partial response. (Reproduced with permission from the authors.)

both infusion-related reactions and IgM flare, both known risks of rituximab in WM, from 59% to 43% and from 47% to 8%, respectively. The PFS advantage of IR versus R plus placebo was seen regardless of genotype and lines of therapy (**Fig. 2**). However, the impressive response rate and PFS seen in the MYD88 WT population should be cautiously interpreted. In iNNOVATE, 16% of the patients randomized to ibrutinib and rituximab who were genotyped were categorized as MYD88 WT, which is at least 2-fold higher than reported in other studies. This discrepancy can be explained by the methodology used to assess MYD88 mutation status; the less-sensitive technique of NGS on unselected bone marrow or paraffin-embedded tissue is associated with higher rates of false-negative results.[10] This study has raised interesting questions in the treatment of WM. How much does the addition of rituximab to ibrutinib differ from ibrutinib alone? Is the finding of responses across CXCR4 mutational status practice changing? Should clinicians who do not have ready access to reliable CXCR4 testing be inclined to add rituximab to ibrutinib since we know that CXCR4-mutated patients carry inherent biologic resistance to ibrutinib? Nonetheless, the iNNOVATE trial clearly underlines the robust clinical activity and tolerance of ibrutinib and rituximab in patients not refractory to rituximab.

The third large trial to include ibrutinib in TN patients with WM is the ASPEN trial, which will be addressed in more detail later in this article. ASPEN is a phase III open-label study comparing ibrutinib to zanubrutinib, a next-generation BTKi, in both TN patients and previously treated patients with WM.[11] Of the 99 patients randomized to ibrutinib, only 18 (18.2%) were treatment naïve. All were MYD88 mutated and 20.2% carried CXCR4 mutations. Despite the small number of previously untreated patients, the study's findings, initially published in 2020 and more recently updated in 2022 (Dimopoulos and colleagues, in press), are very similar to those from Treon and colleagues and from iNNOVATE. Data were reported for all patients (not just treatment naïve) at a median follow-up of 44.4 months; the MRR was 80%, the PFS for all ibrutinib-treated patients was 70% (49% for the CXCR4-mutated patients), 20% discontinued due to AEs, and 27% required a dose reduction of ibrutinib. Adverse effects were also consistent with prior studies whereby 21% of subjects developed any grade atrial fibrillation and 25% any grade hypertension, of which 20% were grade 3 or greater.

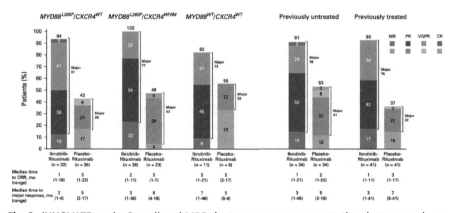

Fig. 2. iNNOVATE study. Overall and MRRs by treatment group, mutational status, and previously treated versus previously untreated patients. CR, complete response; MR, minor response; PR partial response; VGPR, very good partial response. (Reproduced and adapted by permission of the authors.)

What is clear from the limited numbers of patients treated initially with ibrutinib relative to the larger number treated beyond first line is that both the results in terms of efficacy and tolerability are remarkably similar. It is quite legitimate to extrapolate data utilizing ibrutinib beyond first line to TN patients.

More recently, so-called real-world data are emerging concerning the use of front-line ibrutinib in patients with WM. Abeykoon and colleagues from the Mayo Clinic retrospectively identified 13 TN patients treated with ibrutinib monotherapy with a relatively short median follow-up of 19 months.[12] Genotyping information was sporadic and response data were only available for 9 of 13 TN patients: all responded and the MRR was 78%. More recently, Abeykoon and colleagues reported at ASCO 2022 their retrospective experience in 347 TN patients with WM who received chemoimmunotherapy with bendamustine and rituximab (n = 208) or ibrutinib (n = 139) treated between 2011 and 2021. Again, with a median follow-up of 4.2 years, the 4-year PFS was 73% in both groups, although there was a higher VGPR rate in the bendamustine and rituximab group. This study, therefore, corroborates the findings of the smaller prospective studies detailed above.

Zanubrutinib

Zanubrutinib is a second-generation, potent, and more selective irreversible covalent BTKi designed to maximize BTK occupancy and minimize inhibition of off-target kinases, which may be responsible for adverse events typically observed with this class of drugs. The FDA has approved zanubrutinib for patients with relapsed refractory (R/R) mantle cell lymphoma (MCL), patients with marginal zone lymphoma (MZL) who have had at least one anti-CD20–based treatment, patients with WM and with chronic lymphocytic leukemia (CLL). Zanubrutinib has also received EMA approval for WM, MZL, and CLL.

Phase 1/2 study with zanubrutinib in B-cell malignancies
In the first-in-human, multicenter, phase 1/2 study of zanubrutinib in patients with B-cell malignancies (BGB-3111 AU-003),[13] no maximum tolerated dose was identified in part 1, and 160 mg twice daily or 320 mg daily were identified as the recommended phase 2 dose, the former being preferred based on more favorable pharmacodynamic profile with near complete BTK occupancy in lymph nodes. The part 2 of the study included 77 patients with WM, of whom 24 were TN and 53 relapsed/refractory. The primary efficacy endpoint was the rate of VGPR or CR. Of 73 patients evaluable for efficacy, the rate of VGPR or CR was 45% in TN and 51% in R/R patients. The proportion of patients achieving VGPR/CR increased with treatment duration, reaching 44% in TN cohort and 49% in R/R cohort at 24 months. Among 65 patients with available genotype, the VGPR/CR rate was 59%, 27% and 25%, respectively, in patients who were MYD88 (L265P)/CXCR4WT, MYD88 (L265P)/CXCR4WHIM and MYD88 WT.

The median PFS in patients with R/R disease was not reached after a median follow-up of 36.8 months. The estimated event-free rates at 18, 24, and 36 months were 84%, 76%, and 76%, respectively. The median PFS in TN patients was not reached after a median follow-up of 23 months. The estimated event-free rates at 18 and 24 months were both 92%. The estimated 3-year progression-free survival rate was 80.5%, and the overall survival rate was 85%. Adverse events of interest included contusion (32.5%, all grade 1), neutropenia (18%), major hemorrhage (3.9%), atrial fibrillation/flutter (5.2%), and grade 3 diarrhea (2.6%).

The ASPEN study

The randomized open-label multicenter phase III ASPEN trial was designed to compare the efficacy and safety of zanubrutinib with ibrutinib in MYD88 mutated patients with WM.[11] The study included either R/R patients with WM not previously treated with BTK inhibitors, or TN patients unsuitable to standard chemoimmunotherapy. Patients were stratified by CXCR4 status (CXCR4WHIM vs CXCR4WT vs missing) and number of prior lines of therapy (0 vs 1–3 vs > 3). The study included a larger cohort of 201 MYD88 mutated patients (Cohort 1, n = 201) randomized to receive zanubrutinib 160 mg BID or ibrutinib 420 mg once daily (QD), and a smaller cohort of 28 MYD88 WT patients who received zanubrutinib 160 mg *bis in die* (BID) (Cohort 2). Treatment was administered until progression, unacceptable toxicity, death, or withdrawal of consent, whichever occurred first. The study's primary endpoint was the CR or VGPR rate in cohort 1. Key secondary endpoints were MRR, PFS, DOR, OS and safety. The primary endpoint of the study was not met, since by IRC-assessment the CR + VGPR rate was not significantly higher in patients treated with zanubrutinib as compared with patients treated with ibrutinib (28.4% versus 17.2%, $P = .09$). Responses deepened over time and at 44.4 months the CR + VGPR rate reached 36.5% with zanubrutinib and 25.3% with ibrutinib in MYD88 mutated patients, and 30.7% in MYD88 WT patients.[14] In patients with CXCR4 mutation responses were deeper and faster with zanubrutinib than with ibrutinib (VGPR + CR rate 44.6% versus 21.2%, the median time to major response 3.4 months versus 6.6 months). In the single-arm Cohort 2 MYD88 WT patients, the MRR was 50%, including 27% VGPR.[15] At 18 months, PFS was similar in the 2 treatment arms (85% with zanubrutinib versus 84% with ibrutinib).

Zanubrutinib was associated with meaningful advantages in terms of safety and tolerability. In particular, a significantly lower rate of atrial fibrillation was observed in patients treated with zanubrutinib as compared with ibrutinib (3% versus 18%, $P = .0004$). On the other hand, zanubrutinib was associated with a significantly higher rate of neutropenia (32% versus 15%), which did not translate into a higher incidence of infections. With longer follow-up, zanubrutinib confirmed a favorable safety profile, with a significantly lower incidence of adverse events leading to treatment discontinuation or dose reduction. In particular, the cumulative incidence of atrial fibrillation (7.9% versus 23.5%) and hypertension (14.9% versus 25.5%) was significantly lower as compared with ibrutinib.[14] The safety profile of zanubrutinib in patients with WM is consistent with that reported in other B-cell malignancies.[16]

Phase 2 expanded access study (BGB-3111–216)

Fifty patients with WM (17 treatment naïve and 33 relapsed/refractory with a median of 2 earlier therapies) were treated with zanubrutinib 160 BID or 320 mg OD across 10 academic and community medical centers in the United States. Median age was 72 year and most were classified as intermediate (54%) or high-risk (40%) disease. Overall, major, and VGPR were observed in 85%, 73%, and 39% of patients, respectively. Despite older age and high proportion of intermediate-high risk patients, efficacy and safety results were comparable to those reported in ASPEN trial.[17]

Acalabrutinib

Acalabrutinib is a highly selective second-generation irreversible BTK and does not affect other kinases, such as EGFR, Tec, or interleukin-2-inducible kinase, associated with side effects such as rash, atrial fibrillation, or suppression of Natural killer (NK) cell activity. The Food and Drug Administration (FDA) has approved this agent for relapsed or refractory MCL. The safety and efficacy of acalabrutinib in patients with WM was investigated in a phase II study including 106 patients with WM, 92 R/R and 14 TN patients.[18] Patients received 100 mg oral acalabrutinib bid until disease progression or unacceptable toxicity. The study's primary endpoint was the overall response rate (ORR). The ORR was 93% in both groups, with an MRR of 79% in TN patients and 80% in relapsed/refractory patients. In MYD88-mutated patients, the ORR was 94%, including 81% MRR and 11% VGPR. Corresponding response rates in MYD88 wild-type patients were 79%, 64%, and no VGPR or better was observed. PFS at 24 months was, respectively, 90% (95% CI 47.3–98.5) and 81.9% (95% CI 72.1–88.5). CXCR4 mutation status was not assessed in this trial.

At a median follow-up of 27.4 months (range = 4.6–40.7 months), 72% of patients remained on treatment. Treatment discontinuation due to adverse events was 21% in TN patients and 4% in relapsed/refractory patients, respectively. The most common treatment-related adverse events were bleeding (56%) mostly of grade 1 to 2, headache (39%), diarrhea (31%), contusion (29%), and dizziness (25%). Grade 3/4 neutropenia was observed in 16% of patients. Atrial fibrillation occurred in 3% of patients.

Tirabrutinib

Tirabrutinib is a second-generation, irreversible, BTKi that was approved in 2020 for the treatment of patients with WM in Japan, based on the results of a multicenter, open-label, single-arm, phase II study (ONO-4059–05) including 27 patients, 18 not previously treated and 9 who had received one or more systemic treatment.[19] Patients received tirabrutinib orally at a daily dose of 480 mg under fasting conditions until disease progression or unacceptable toxicity. MRR was 93%, including a VGPR + CR rate of 22% after the primary analysis. In an updated analysis, with a median follow-up of 24.8 months, the PFS and OS rates at 24 months were 92.6% and 100%, respectively. Treatment-related skin adverse events were observed in 52% of patients. Bleeding was reported in 33% of patients (all grade 1–2), whereas atrial fibrillation and hypertension were reported in 4% of patients each.

Zanubrutinib in Patients Intolerant to Ibrutinib or Acalabrutinib

A phase 2, multicenter, open-label, single-arm study conducted in the United States investigated treatment with zanubrutinib in 67 patients with CLL/small lymphocytic lymphoma, MCL, WM, or MZL who became intolerant to ibrutinib, acalabrutinib, or both. The primary endpoint was recurrence and change in severity of ibrutinib or acalabrutinib intolerance events based on investigator-assessed adverse events. Most intolerance events (70% for ibrutinib and 83% for acalabrutinib) did not recur with zanubrutinib. Of the recurring events, 79% of ibrutinib intolerance events and 33% of acalabrutinib intolerance event recurred at a lower severity with zanubrutinib. Moreover, no events recurred at higher severity. These data suggest that zanubrutinib may represent a viable treatment option for patients intolerant to ibrutinib and/or acalabrutinib.[20]

Withdrawal Syndrome and IgM Rebound after Discontinuation of BTK Inhibitors

Clinicians must be aware of the possible onset of withdrawal symptoms including fever, pain, and fatigue following interruption of BTK inhibitors, which is sometimes needed to manage toxicities or perioperatively to reduce the risk of bleeding. Symptoms have been reported to occur in about 20% of patients with WM who hold ibrutinib, generally within 2 days of hold, and resolve rapidly after reinitiation of therapy. Steroids may be useful to control withdrawal symptoms while waiting to resume treatment.[21]

Discontinuation of BTK inhibitors may also be followed by an IgM rebound that was reported in 25% of patients at 3 weeks and 65% at 5 weeks. The IgM rebound is normally asymptomatic but sometimes may be abrupt and complicated by hyperviscosity syndrome requiring emergent plasmapheresis. For those patients with progression, timely initiation of salvage therapy diminishes the risk of IgM rebound.[22,23]

BTK Inhibitors as Primary Therapy for Waldenström Macroglobulinemia

There are no published prospective randomized studies comparing efficacy and safety of BTK inhibitors with chemoimmunotherapy, which has been considered the standard frontline approach in the past 2 decades, until BTK inhibitors became available. The ongoing RAINBOW trial (NCT04061512) is comparing rituximab-ibrutinib with dexamethasone–rituximab-cyclophosphamide. Furthermore, data on the optimal sequencing of available therapies are currently limited to a single retrospective study showing comparable outcomes of patients receiving chemoimmunotherapy frontline and BTK inhibitors at first relapse as compared with patients treated with the opposite sequencing (Tawqif and colleagues.[24] EHA 2022). While waiting to get more evidence on the best sequencing, the choice between BTK inhibitors or chemoimmunotherapy frontline is mainly driven by patients' characteristics (age, fitness, comorbidities) and practical considerations (indefinite oral versus fixed-duration parenteral therapy, costs, and drug reimbursement). A therapeutic algorithm based on genomic profile was proposed some years ago, indicating ibrutinib as the first-choice for MYD88-mutated/CXCR4 wild-type patients and for MYD88-mutated/CXCR4-mutated patients for whom a rapid response is not needed, whereas chemoimmunotherapy was considered the preferred option in MYD88-mutated/CXCR4-mutated patients in need of a rapid response and in MYD88 wild-type subjects.[25] However, this scenario has changed with the approval of second-generation BTKi zanubrutinib, which has demonstrated remarkable activity also in CXCR4-mutated patients and in MYD88 wild-type ones.

Preliminary data from retrospective studies suggest that TP53 aberrations are associated with chemoresistance in WM,[26] as in other lymphoproliferative disorders. With the availability of an alternative to chemotherapy, these abnormalities could become relevant as a driver of treatment choice in the next future.

SUMMARY

BTK inhibitors have demonstrated clinically meaningful efficacy in patients with previously untreated WM. In a head-to-head comparison with ibrutinib, zanubrutinib was not significantly superior to ibrutinib but provided faster and deeper response in CXCR4-mutated patients. Furthermore, unlike ibrutinib, second-generation BTK inhibitors acalabrutinib and zanubrutinib showed activity also in MYD88 WT patients.

The safety advantages of second-generation BTK inhibitors are consistent with less off-target activity compared with ibrutinib. In a head-to-head comparison with ibrutinib, fewer adverse events leading to treatment discontinuation, dose reductions, and deaths occurred in the zanubrutinib arm. The cumulative incidences of atrial fibrillation, diarrhea, and hypertension were lower in patients receiving zanubrutinib. Despite a higher rate of neutropenia in the zanubrutinib arm, infection rates were similar. Real-world data are eagerly awaited to confirm the efficacy and safety of BTK inhibitors in unselected patients with WM.

CLINICS CARE POINTS

- BTK inhibitors are highly effective and well tolerated as front-line treatment of WM.

- Clinical responses to BTK inhibitors are influenced by both MYD88 and CXCR4 mutational status.
- Complete response is quite rare with BTK inhibitors, despite their robust clinical activity.
- In selected situations, there are data supporting adding rituximab to ibrutinib.
- The next-generation BTK inhibitors have fewer off-target effects because of their higher selectivity compared with ibrutinib.
- While BTK inhibitors have a well-established role in patients relapsing after chemoimmunotherapy, evidence in the frontline setting is more limited. Studies comparing BTK inhibitors with chemoimmunotherapy in TN patients with WM are ongoing and will determine whether BTK inhibitors should be considered the standard of care for all or for definite subsets of patients.

DISCLOSURE

M. Varettoni: ABBVIE: advisory board, speaker honoraria; AstraZeneca: advisory board, speaker honoraria; Beigene: advisory board; Janssen: advisory board.J.V. Matous: Beigene: advisory board; Janssen: advisory board.

REFERENCES

1. Treon SP, Xu L, Yang G, et al. MYD88 L265P Somatic Mutation in Waldenström's Macroglobulinemia. N Engl J Med 2012;367(9):826–33.
2. Treon SP, Tripsas CK, Meid K, et al. Ibrutinib in Previously Treated Waldenström's Macroglobulinemia. N Engl J Med 2015;372(15):1430–40.
3. Treon SP, Meid K, Gustine J, et al. Long-Term Follow-Up of Ibrutinib Monotherapy in Symptomatic, Previously Treated Patients With Waldenström Macroglobulinemia. J Clin Oncol 2021;39(6):565–75.
4. Dimopoulos MA, Trotman J, Tedeschi A, et al. Ibrutinib for patients with rituximab-refractory Waldenström's macroglobulinaemia (iNNOVATE): an open-label substudy of an international, multicentre, phase 3 trial. The Lancet oncology 2017; 18(2):241–50.
5. Treon SP, Gustine J, Meid K, et al. Ibrutinib Monotherapy in Symptomatic, Treatment Naïve Patients With Waldenström Macroglobulinemia. J Clin Oncol 2018; 36(27):2755–61.
6. Castillo JJ, Meid K, Gustine JN, et al. Long-term follow-up of ibrutinib monotherapy in treatment-naive patients with Waldenstrom macroglobulinemia. Leukemia 2022;36(2):532–9.
7. Castillo JJ, Xu L, Gustine JN, et al. CXCR4 mutation subtypes impact response and survival outcomes in patients with Waldenström macroglobulinaemia treated with ibrutinib. Br J Haematol 2019;187(3):356–63.
8. Dimopoulos MA, Tedeschi A, Trotman J, et al. Phase 3 Trial of Ibrutinib plus Rituximab in Waldenström's Macroglobulinemia. N Engl J Med 2018;378(25): 2399–410.
9. Buske C, Tedeschi A, Trotman J, et al. Ibrutinib Plus Rituximab Versus Placebo Plus Rituximab for Waldenström's Macroglobulinemia: Final Analysis From the Randomized Phase III iNNOVATE Study. J Clin Oncol 2022;40(1):52–62.
10. Kofides A, Hunter ZR, Xu L, et al. Diagnostic Next-generation Sequencing Frequently Fails to Detect MYD88(L265P) in Waldenström Macroglobulinemia. Hemasphere 2021;5(8):e624.

11. Tam CS, Opat S, D'Sa S, et al. A randomized phase 3 trial of zanubrutinib vs ibrutinib in symptomatic Waldenström macroglobulinemia: the ASPEN study. Blood 2020;136(18):2038–50.
12. Abeykoon JP, Zanwar S, Ansell SM, et al. Ibrutinib monotherapy outside of clinical trial setting in Waldenström macroglobulinaemia: practice patterns, toxicities and outcomes. Br J Haematol 2020;188(3):394–403.
13. Trotman J, Opat S, Gottlieb D, et al. Zanubrutinib for the treatment of patients with Waldenström macroglobulinemia: 3 years of follow-up. Blood 2020;136(18): 2027–37.
14. Tam CS, Garcia-Sanz R, Opat S, et al. ASPEN: Long-term follow-up results of a phase 3 randomized trial of zanubrutinib (ZANU) versus ibrutinib (IBR) in patients with Waldenström macroglobulinemia (WM). J Clin Oncol 2022;40(16_suppl): 7521.
15. Dimopoulos M, Sanz RG, Lee H-P, et al. Zanubrutinib for the treatment of MYD88 wild-type Waldenström macroglobulinemia: a substudy of the phase 3 ASPEN trial. Blood Adv 2020;4(23):6009–18.
16. Tam CS, Dimopoulos M, Garcia-Sanz R, et al. Pooled safety analysis of zanubrutinib monotherapy in patients with B-cell malignancies. Blood Adv 2022;6(4): 1296–308.
17. Castillo JJ, Kingsley EC, Narang M, et al. Zanubrutinib in patients with treatment-naïve or relapsed/refractory Waldenström macroglobulinemia: An expanded-access study of 50 patients in the United States. EJHaem 2023;4(1):301–4.
18. Owen RG, McCarthy H, Rule S, et al. Acalabrutinib monotherapy in patients with Waldenström macroglobulinemia: a single-arm, multicentre, phase 2 study. Lancet Haematol 2020;7(2):e112–21.
19. Sekiguchi N, Rai S, Munakata W, et al. A multicenter, open-label, phase II study of tirabrutinib (ONO/GS-4059) in patients with Waldenström's macroglobulinemia. Cancer Sci 2020;111(9):3327–37.
20. Shadman M, Flinn IW, Levy MY, et al. Zanubrutinib in patients with previously treated B-cell malignancies intolerant of previous Bruton tyrosine kinase inhibitors in the USA: a phase 2, open-label, single-arm study. Lancet Haematol 2023; 10(1):e35–45.
21. Castillo JJ, Gustine JN, Meid K, et al. Ibrutinib withdrawal symptoms in patients with Waldenström macroglobulinemia. Haematologica 2018;103:e308.
22. Gustine JN, Meid K, Dubeau T, et al. Ibrutinib discontinuation in Waldenström macroglobulinemia: Etiologies, outcomes, and IgM rebound. Am J Hematol 2018;93(4):511–7.
23. Gustine JN, Sarosiek S, Flinn CA, et al. Natural history of Waldenström macroglobulinemia following acquired resistance to ibrutinib monotherapy. Haematologica 2022;107(5):1163–71.
24. Tawfiq R, Abeykoon J, Zanwar S, Paludo J, Kapoor P. Outcomes and treatment patterns after first relapse in patients with waldenström macroglobulinemia. HemaSphere 2022;6(S3):1991.
25. Castillo JJ, Treon SP. Management of Waldenström macroglobulinemia in 2020. Hematology Am Soc Hematol Educ Program 2020;2020(1):372–9.
26. Poulain S, Roumier C, Bertrand E, et al. TP53 Mutation and Its Prognostic Significance in Waldenstrom's macroglobulinemia. Clin Cancer Res 2017;23(20): 6325–35.

Future Directions in the Frontline Management of Waldenström Macroglobulinemia

Christian Buske, MD[a],*, Maria Lia Palomba, MD[b]

KEYWORDS

- Waldenstrom's macroglobulinemia • Treatment-naïve • Chemoimmunotherapy
- BTK-inhibitors • Front-line

KEY POINTS

- The ultimate goal of future front-line treatments for Waldenström macroglobulinemia (WM) is to develop therapies that can induce complete remissions, translating into long disease-free intervals and, by this, approaching functional cure in the mostly elderly patient population.
- Future front-line treatments need to be well tolerated and should guarantee a good quality of life in WM, which is indolent in nature and often affects patients with age-associated comorbidities.
- The development of fixed-duration treatment concepts is of high importance as it will ensure better tolerability for the patients and also better cost-effectiveness.
- Future frontline treatments should be accessible worldwide and not limited to Western industrialized countries.

ASYMPTOMATIC PATIENTS

Newly diagnosed Waldenström macroglobulinemia (WM) patients with no significant cytopenias, normal organ functions, and no WM-related symptoms such as hyperviscosity or peripheral neuropathy (smoldering WM) can be safely observed expectantly without compromising their overall survival (OS). Initiation of therapy is contemplated when patients become symptomatic or when hematologic or organ function parameters become significantly altered. Identifying a serum immunoglobin M (IgM) level greater than 4500 mg/dL, greater than 70% bone marrow involvement by lymphoplasmacytic lymphoma (LPL), beta-2 microglobulin greater than 4 mg/dL, and serum albumin less than 3.5 g/dL at diagnosis portends a higher risk of disease progression

[a] University Hospital Ulm, Institute for Experimental Cancer Research, Albert – Einstein Allee 11, Ulm 89081, Germany; [b] Memorial Sloan Kettering Cancer Center, 1275 York Avenue, New York, NY 10065, USA
* Corresponding author.
E-mail address: christian.buske@uni-ulm.de

Hematol Oncol Clin N Am 37 (2023) 719–725
https://doi.org/10.1016/j.hoc.2023.05.001
0889-8588/23/© 2023 Elsevier Inc. All rights reserved.

requiring therapy initiation.[1] A model using those parameters identified three risk groups with a median time to progression (TTP) varying between 1.8 and 9.3 years. Furthermore, MYD88 wild-type disease had significantly shorter TTP. This confirms previous evidence that patients with wild-type *MYD88* have more aggressive disease and share genomic alterations with diffuse large B-cell lymphoma (DLBCL).[2–4] Somatic mutations in the C-terminal domain of *CXCR4*, which occur in about 40% of WM,[5] can also affect disease presentation. *CXCR4*-mutated WM tends to have higher serum IgM levels, more bone marrow (BM) infiltration, less nodal involvement field 6, and partial resistance to ibrutinib alone.[6,7] Resistance to zanubrutinib and ixazomib has also been linked to *CXCR4* mutated status.[8,9] Given what we now understand about the existence of WM with distinct prognosis and response to therapy, it is intuitive to ask whether patients with a high risk of early progression or transformation to DLBCL would benefit from early intervention. Ultimately, single cell and immune signatures of tumor evolution in patients with newly diagnosed WM at risk for early progression might shape treatment decisions regarding timing and type of first-line therapy. However, a watch-and-wait approach to WM remains the preferred choice for asymptomatic WM patients.

PATIENTS IN NEED OF TREATMENT

Once indications for treatment initiation are met, the choice of initial therapy requires as much knowledge of each patient's genetic and genomic data as is feasible at the center where the patient is being treated, with the understanding that this information might not be readily available in smaller nonacademic centers.[10] A list of therapy options for treatment-naïve WM is shown in **Table 1**. Except for rituximab monotherapy, all regimens listed provide major response rates (at least partial response [PR]) of 67% or higher, up to 88% in the case of rituximab–bendamustine, versus 40% for rituximab alone. Yet, the rate of very good PR [VGPR] (>90% reduction of IgM levels from baseline, VGPR) is in most cases in the 20% to 35% and often in the single-digit range. Rates of complete response (CR; defined as normal IgM level and complete absence of paraprotein by immunofixation) are rarer and often not achieved at any line of therapy, even with long follow-up and despite achieving deepening of response over time. The lack of satisfactory CR rates observed in WM indicates the presence of subclones with intrinsic drug resistance, for instance, by maintaining IRAK1/IRAK4 activity despite suppression of Bruton Tyrosine Kinase (BTK) or by the emergence of mutated BTK or downstream members of the B-cell receptor (BCR) pathway, as in the case of ibrutinib.[11–14] The persistence of CD20-positive plasma cells is another reason for persistent paraprotein production, even in the total absence of LPL cells in posttreatment biopsies.[15] Attainment of CR matters because, as shown in rituximab monotherapy, it is associated with longer progression-free survival,[16] though it is unclear whether it impacts OS. Intuitively, a combinatorial approach to lymphoma cell survival pathways is the optimal tactic to eradicate the WM clone, obtain higher rates of CRs, and hopefully limit the duration of therapy and extend responses. As single agents, all BTKis require continued exposure for the disease to remain in check.

EMERGING TREATMENTS

There are several new classes of drugs being currently tested in relapsed/refractory WM, which have the potential to move to first-line treatment soon and, with this, to change the treatment landscape for treatment naïve patients with this lymphoma subtype. The non-covalent BTK inhibitor pirtobrutinib has shown remarkable activity in WM patients who failed treatment with covalent BTK inhibitors (cBTKis), mostly

Table 1
Selected data from prospective studies in treatment-naïve patients with Waldenström macroglobulinemia

Study	Regimen	N	PR or Better	VGPR or Better	PFS
Dimopoulos et al,[26] 2007 Kastritis et al,[27] 2015	Dexamethasone Rituximab Cyclophosphamide	72	74%	7%	35 mo (median)
Rummel et al,[28] 2013	Bendamustine Rituximab	257	88%	4%	65 mo (median)
Treon et al,[29] 2009 Treon et al,[30] 2015	Bortezomib Dexamethasone Rituximab	23	83%	35%	66 mo (median)
Dimopoulos et al,[31] 2013 Gavriatopoulou et al,[32] 2017	Bortezomib weekly Dexamethasone Rituximab	59	68%	10%	42 mo (median)
Treon et al,[33] 2014	Carfilzomib Dexamethasone Rituximab	28	68%	36%	46 mo (median)
Castillo et al,[9] 2018 Castillo et al,[34] 2020	Ixazomib Dexamethasone Rituximab	26	77%	19%	40 mo (median)
Buske et al,[35] 2023	Bortezomib Cyclophosphamide Dexamethasone Rituximab	102	81%	17%	81% at 24 mo
	Cyclophosphamide Dexamethasone Rituximab	100	70%	10%	73% at 24 months
Treon et al,[36] 2018 Castillo et al,[37] 2022	Ibrutinib	30	87%	30%	76% at 4 y
Dimopoulos et al,[38] 2018 Buske et al,[7] 2022	Ibrutinib Rituximab	34	76%	27%	70% at 4.5 y
	Rituximab	34	41%	9%	32% at 4.5 y
Tam et al,[8] 2020	Zanubrutinib	19	74%	36%	78% at 42 mo
	Ibrutinib	18	67%	22%	70% at 42 mo
Owen et al,[39] 2020	Acalabrutinib	14	79%	NR	86% at 66 mo

Abbreviations: N, number of patients; NR, not reported; PFS, progression-free survival; PR, partial response; VGPR, very good partial response.
Adapted from Ref.[25]

ibrutinib, in the large Phase 1/2 Bruin trial program. In this trial, pirtobrutinib induced a 66.7% overall response rate in 63 patients previously exposed to cBTKis, with nearly 25% achieving a CR/VGPR and a median PFS of 19.4 months. This encouraging activity was accompanied by an excellent toxicity profile with a very low frequency of ≥ grade 3 events except for neutropenia.[17] Of note, ≥ grade 3 hypertension and atrial fibrillation occurred in only 2.3% and 1.2% of patients. The BCL2 inhibitor venetoclax has been successfully tested in relapsed/refractory WM in a single arm phase II study; 32 evaluable patients were treated until progression or intolerable side effects. Venetoclax induced a major response rate of 81% and CR/VGPR of 19% with a PFS of 30 months. Of note, activity seemed to be independent of the *CXCR4* mutational status. These data established venetoclax as an attractive compound for the first-line treatment of WM. However, the challenge is that despite their encouraging clinical activity, pirtobrutinib and venetoclax as single agents remain a non-fixed duration treatment, similar to the cBTKi. This is a major disadvantage of those emerging treatment concepts inducing cumulative toxicity over time, challenging the patient's compliance, and ultimately causing a substantial financial burden. Thus, there is consensus that the future direction of treatments, particularly in the first-line setting, must move to time-limited treatment.

THE VISION OF FUTURE FRONT-LINE TREATMENT IN WALDENSTRÖM MACROGLOBULINEMIA

Current options for front-line treatment are mainly chemotherapy-based or non-fixed duration, chemotherapy-free cBTKi therapies. How to move on from here? There is consensus that further dose intensification of conventional immunochemotherapy will most likely not succeed and would result in unacceptable toxicity in the mostly elderly population of WM patients. Thus, targeted treatment approaches exemplified by the class of BTKi or venetoclax will potentially act as the backbone of future combination regimens. The next major goal will be to overcome their major limitation of indefinite—duration application. Realistically, this goal will be achieved soon as targeted treatment concepts with different modes of action are already available or tested as single agents in clinical trials. The next logical step to combine these agents, and by doing so to establish chemo-free concepts applied for a defined period, is on the way. In a phase II trial, ibrutinib was combined with venetoclax in 45 treatment naïve WM patients for up to 2 years. Efficacy was impressive, with a 100% overall response rate and 93% major response rate with a short time to major response of 1.9 months. However, the study was prematurely stopped because of unforeseen cardiac toxicity with one grade 4 and two fatal ventricular arrythmia.[18] This illustrates that new combinations must be carefully tested in prospective clinical trials to confirm their feasibility in WM and that we should not extrapolate safety data from related lymphoma subtypes to WM. Toxicity in this trial might result from known off-target effects of ibrutinib. Future trials must confirm that a combination of second-generation cBTKi, such as zanubrutinib or non-covalent BTKi, such as pirtobrutinib, is safe when combined with venetoclax. The combination of venetoclax/rituximab (Ven-R) was highly effective and safe in chronic lymphocytic leukemia.[19] The European Consortium for Waldenström Macroglobulinemia is planning a randomized phase II study comparing 12 months of treatment with Ven-R versus Dexamethasone, Rituximab, Cyclophosphamide (DRC) for six cycles in treatment naïve WM (ClinicalTrials.gov identifier: NCT05099471). In this trial, a timely fixed-duration chemo-free approach is compared with standard immunochemotherapy for the first time, which will help to reevaluate the role of rituximab/chemotherapy in the era of targeted treatments in WM.

Despite these new developments, innovative treatment concepts beyond BTK or BCL2 inhibition are needed. Exciting data about bi-specific anti-CD20/CD3 antibodies were reported in various related B-cell lymphomas, such as follicular lymphoma, DLBCL, and mantle cell lymphoma. These bi-specific antibodies induced deep remissions and encouraging durable remissions in heavily pretreated and refractory patients and are currently tested as single agents or in combination regimens in a variety of clinical trials.[20,21] Chimeric antigen receptor-T cell (CAR-T) cells, retrovirally engineered autologous T cells programmed to attack CD19-positive B cells, have shown tremendous efficacy in relapsed/refractory DLBCL and in follicular lymphoma.[22,23] Studies for both immunotherapy classes are planned or ongoing in WM. These two examples, bi-specific antibodies and CAR-T cells, demonstrate that rapid progress has been made in developing innovative treatment concepts which engage the patient's immune system. Data for these approaches in WM are still very limited, and no data exist in treatment naïve WM patients.[24] However, it is conceivable that bi-specific antibodies might move to front-line treatment in WM if data in the relapsed/refractory setting are comparable to their efficacy in follicular lymphoma. Taking it all together, hope is justified that we can offer well-tolerated and highly efficient targeted treatments of fixed-time duration to treatment naïve WM patients shortly, avoiding chemotherapy-associated toxicity and being able to induce functional cure in most WM patients.

AUTHOR DISCLOSURES

C. Buske received honoraria from Roche, Pfizer, Janssen, Hexal, Celltrion, AbbVie, Novartis, Bayer, Morphosys, Regeneron, Beigene; consulting fees from Roche, Pfizer, Janssen, Hexal, Celltrion, AbbVie, Novartis, Bayer, Morphosys, Regeneron, Beigene, Sobi; and Research Funding from Roche, Switzerland, Janssen, United States, Celltrion, South Korea, AbbVie, United States, Bayer, United States, Amgen, United States, and MSD. M.L. Palomba received honoraria from BMS, Kite, Synthekine, and Cellectar.

REFERENCES

1. Bustoros M, Sklavenitis-Pistofidis R, Kapoor P, et al. Progression risk stratification of asymptomatic Waldenström macroglobulinemia. J Clin Oncol 2019;37(16): 1403–11.
2. Treon SP, Gustine J, Xu L, et al. MYD88 wild-type Waldenstrom Macroglobulinaemia: differential diagnosis, risk of histological transformation, and overall survival. Br J Haematol 2018;180(3):374–80.
3. Treon SP, Xu L, Hunter Z. MYD88 Mutations and Response to Ibrutinib in Waldenström's Macroglobulinemia. N Engl J Med 2015;373(6):584–6.
4. Varettoni M, Zibellini S, Arcaini L, et al. MYD88 (L265P) mutation is an independent risk factor for progression in patients with IgM monoclonal gammopathy of undetermined significance. Blood 2013;122(13):2284–5.
5. Hunter ZR, Xu L, Yang G, et al. The genomic landscape of Waldenstrom macroglobulinemia is characterized by highly recurring MYD88 and WHIM-like CXCR4 mutations, and small somatic deletions associated with B-cell lymphomagenesis. Blood 2014;123(11):1637–46.
6. Treon SP, Tripsas CK, Meid K, et al. Ibrutinib in previously treated Waldenstrom's macroglobulinemia. N Engl J Med 2015;372(15):1430–40.
7. Buske C, Tedeschi A, Trotman J, et al. Ibrutinib plus rituximab versus placebo plus rituximab for Waldenstrom's macroglobulinemia: final analysis from the randomized phase III iNNOVATE study. J Clin Oncol 2022;40(1):52–62.
8. Tam CS, Opat S, D'Sa S, et al. A randomized phase 3 trial of zanubrutinib vs ibrutinib in symptomatic Waldenstrom macroglobulinemia: the ASPEN study. Blood 2020;136(18):2038–50.
9. Castillo JJ, Meid K, Gustine JN, et al. Prospective clinical trial of ixazomib, dexamethasone, and rituximab as primary therapy in waldenstrom macroglobulinemia. Clin Cancer Res 2018;24(14):3247–52.
10. Treon SP, Xu L, Guerrera ML, et al. Genomic landscape of Waldenstrom macroglobulinemia and its impact on treatment strategies. J Clin Oncol 2020;38(11): 1198–208.
11. Yang G, Zhou Y, Liu X, et al. Disruption of MYD88 Pathway signaling leads to loss of constitutive IRAK1, NF-{kappa}{beta} and JAK/STAT signaling and induces

apoptosis of cells expressing the MYD88 L265P mutation in waldenstrom's macroglobulinemia. ASH Annual Meeting Abstracts. November 18, 2011 2011; 118(21):597-.

12. Yang G, Zhou Y, Liu X, et al. A mutation in MYD88 (L265P) supports the survival of lymphoplasmacytic cells by activation of Bruton tyrosine kinase in Waldenstrom macroglobulinemia. Blood 2013;122(7):1222-32.

13. Xu L, Tsakmaklis N, Yang G, et al. Acquired mutations associated with ibrutinib resistance in Waldenstrom macroglobulinemia. Blood 2017;129(18):2519-25.

14. Chen JG, Liu X, Munshi M, et al. BTK(Cys481Ser) drives ibrutinib resistance via ERK1/2 and protects BTK(wild-type) MYD88-mutated cells by a paracrine mechanism. Blood 2018;131(18):2047-59.

15. Barakat FH, Medeiros LJ, Wei EX, et al. Residual monotypic plasma cells in patients with waldenstrom macroglobulinemia after therapy. Am J Clin Pathol 2011; 135(3):365-73.

16. Treon SP, Hanzis C, Manning RJ, et al. Maintenance Rituximab is associated with improved clinical outcome in rituximab naive patients with Waldenstrom Macroglobulinaemia who respond to a rituximab-containing regimen. Br J Haematol 2011;154(3):357-62.

17. Palomba ML, Patel MR, Eyre TA, et al. Efficacy of Pirtobrutinib, a Highly Selective, Non-Covalent (Reversible) BTK Inhibitor in Relapsed/Refractory Waldenström Macroglobulinemia: results from the Phase 1/2 BRUIN Study. Blood 2022; 140(Supplement 1). 5578-560.

18. Castillo JJ, Sarosiek S, Branagan AR, et al. Ibrutinib and venetoclax in previously untreated waldenström macroglobulinemia. Blood 2022;140(Suppl 1):564-5.

19. Kater AP, Wu JQ, Kipps T, et al. Venetoclax plus rituximab in relapsed chronic lymphocytic leukemia: 4-year results and evaluation of impact of genomic complexity and gene mutations from the MURANO phase III study. J Clin Oncol 2020;38(34):4042-54.

20. Buske C. Mosunetuzumab, a bispecific antibody, in patients with relapsed or refractory follicular lymphoma. Lancet Oncol 2022;23(8):967-9.

21. Budde LE, Sehn LH, Matasar M, et al. Safety and efficacy of mosunetuzumab, a bispecific antibody, in patients with relapsed or refractory follicular lymphoma: a single-arm, multicentre, phase 2 study. Lancet Oncol 2022;23(8):1055-65.

22. Albanyan O, Chavez J, Munoz J. The role of CAR-T cell therapy as second line in diffuse large B-cell lymphoma. Ther Adv Hematol 2022;13. https://doi.org/10.1177/20406207221141511. 20406207221141511.

23. Fowler NH, Dickinson M, Dreyling M, et al. Tisagenlecleucel in adult relapsed or refractory follicular lymphoma: the phase 2 ELARA trial. Nat Med 2022;28(2): 325-32.

24. Palomba ML, Qualls D, Monette S, et al. CD19-directed chimeric antigen receptor T cell therapy in Waldenström macroglobulinemia: a preclinical model and initial clinical experience. J Immunother Cancer 2022;10(2). https://doi.org/10.1136/jitc-2021-004128.

25. Buske C, Castillo JJ, Abeykoon JP, et al. Report of consensus panel 1 from the 11th International Workshop on Waldenstrom's Macroglobulinemia on management of symptomatic, treatment-naïve patients. Semin Hematol 2023. https://doi.org/10.1053/j.seminhematol.2023.03.005.

26. Dimopoulos MA, Anagnostopoulos A, Kyrtsonis MC, et al. Primary treatment of Waldenstrom macroglobulinemia with dexamethasone, rituximab, and cyclophosphamide. J Clin Oncol 2007;25(22):3344-9.

27. Kastritis E, Gavriatopoulou M, Kyrtsonis MC, et al. Dexamethasone, rituximab, and cyclophosphamide as primary treatment of Waldenstrom macroglobulinemia: final analysis of a phase 2 study. Blood 2015;126(11):1392–4.
28. Rummel MJ, Niederle N, Maschmeyer G, et al. Bendamustine plus rituximab versus CHOP plus rituximab as first-line treatment for patients with indolent and mantle-cell lymphomas: an open-label, multicentre, randomised, phase 3 non-inferiority trial. Lancet 2013;381(9873):1203–10.
29. Treon SP, Ioakimidis L, Soumerai JD, et al. Primary therapy of Waldenstrom macroglobulinemia with bortezomib, dexamethasone, and rituximab: WMCTG clinical trial 05-180. Clinical Trial Multicenter Study Research Support, N.I.H., Extramural Research Support, Non-U.S. Gov't. J Clin Oncol 2009;27(23):3830–5.
30. Leblebjian H, Noonan K, Paba-Prada C, et al. Cyclophosphamide, bortezomib, and dexamethasone combination in waldenstrom macroglobulinemia. Am J Hematol 2015;90(6):E122–3.
31. Dimopoulos MA, Garcia-Sanz R, Gavriatopoulou M, et al. Primary therapy of Waldenstrom macroglobulinemia (WM) with weekly bortezomib, low-dose dexamethasone, and rituximab (BDR): long-term results of a phase 2 study of the European Myeloma Network (EMN). Blood 2013;122(19):3276–82. https://doi.org/10.1182/blood-2013-05-503862.
32. Gavriatopoulou M, Garcia-Sanz R, Kastritis E, et al. BDR in newly diagnosed patients with WM: final analysis of a phase 2 study after a minimum follow-up of 6 years. Blood 2017;129(4):456–9.
33. Treon SP, Tripsas CK, Meid K, et al. Carfilzomib, rituximab, and dexamethasone (CaRD) treatment offers a neuropathy-sparing approach for treating Waldenstrom's macroglobulinemia. Blood 2014;124(4):503–10.
34. Castillo JJ, Meid K, Flynn CA, et al. Ixazomib, dexamethasone, and rituximab in treatment-naive patients with Waldenstrom macroglobulinemia: long-term follow-up. Blood Adv 2020;4(16):3952–9.
35. Buske C, Dimopoulos MA, Grunenberg A, et al. Bortezomib-dexamethasone, rituximab, and cyclophosphamide as first-line treatment for waldenström's macroglobulinemia: a prospectively randomized trial of the european consortium for waldenström's macroglobulinemia. Journal of Clinical Oncology 2023;Jco2201805. https://doi.org/10.1200/jco.22.01805.
36. Treon SP, Gustine J, Meid K, et al. Ibrutinib monotherapy in symptomatic, treatment-naive patients with waldenstrom macroglobulinemia. J Clin Oncol 2018;36(27):2755–61.
37. Castillo JJ, Meid K, Gustine JN, et al. Long-term follow-up of ibrutinib monotherapy in treatment-naive patients with Waldenstrom macroglobulinemia. Leukemia 2022;36(2):532–9.
38. Dimopoulos MA, Tedeschi A, Trotman J, et al. Phase 3 trial of ibrutinib plus rituximab in Waldenstrom's macroglobulinemia. N Engl J Med 2018;378(25):2399–410.
39. Owen RG, McCarthy H, Rule S, et al. Acalabrutinib monotherapy in patients with Waldenstrom macroglobulinemia: a single-arm, multicentre, phase 2 study. Lancet Haematol 2020;7(2):e112–21.

The Management of Relapsed or Refractory Waldenström's Macroglobulinemia

Ramón García-Sanz, MD, PhD[a,b,*], Alessandra Tedeschi, MD[a,b]

KEYWORDS

- Waldenström's macroglobulinemia • Salvage therapy • Chemoimmunotherapy
- Bruton tyrosine kinase inhibitors

KEY POINTS

- In Waldenström's Macroglobulinemia, the cure is still an unmet challenge.
- Combinations with alkylating agents and/or purine analogs and monoclonal antibodies, Bruton's tyrosine kinase inhibitors, and proteasome inhibitors, are treatment possibilities for relapsed and refractory patients.
- New additional agents can be seen on the horizon as potential effective therapies, including new BTK inhibitors, BCL2 inhibitors, radioconjugated drugs, and CAR T-cells.
- The best therapy in the 2nd line and beyond in Waldenström's Macroglobulinemia patients depends on the prior therapies and their results in terms of effectiveness and toxicity.

INTRODUCTION

The current consensus in Waldenström's macroglobulinemia (WM) states that diagnosis requires the following criteria: the presence of infiltration of clonal lymphoplasmacytic cells documented by bone marrow (BM) biopsy (lymphoplasmacytic lymphoma, LPL) and presence of serum monoclonal immunoglobulin M (IgM), irrespective of M-protein size.[1,2] However, fifth WHO classification still defines IgM monoclonal gammopathy of undetermined significance (IgM-MGUS) by the presence of a serum IgM paraprotein below 30 g/L, BM lymphoplasmacytic infiltration <10%,

[a] Department of Hematology, University Hospital of Salamanca, Research Biomedical Institute of Salamanca (IBSAL), Accelerator Project, Centro de Investigación Biomédica en Red-Cáncer (CIBERONC) CB16/12/00369 and Center for Cancer Research-IBMCC (USAL-CSIC), Paseo de San Vicente, 58-182, Salamanca 37007, Spain; [b] Department of Hematology, Niguarda Cancer Center, ASST Grande Ospedale Metropolitano Niguarda, Milano, Italy
* Corresponding author. Department of Hematology, University Hospital of Salamanca, Building I-J, Floor 3, Laboratory of HLA and molecular biology, Paseo de San Vicente, 58-182, Salamanca 37007, Spain.
E-mail address: rgarcias@usal.es

Hematol Oncol Clin N Am 37 (2023) 727–749
https://doi.org/10.1016/j.hoc.2023.04.006
0889-8588/23/© 2023 Elsevier Inc. All rights reserved.

and no evidence of end-organ damage related to the underlying lymphoproliferative disorder.[3] Both classifications stress the importance of the mutational landscape in WM, especially because genomics greatly impact the response to several therapies.

WM was considered as an intermediate step between mutated chronic lymphocytic leukemia (B-CLL) and multiple myeloma (MM), but the discovery of the $MYD88^{L265P}$ mutation[4] contributed to separation of these entities.[5] The estimated incidence of WM is 3.6 to 5.5 cases per million person-years at risk in Europe and the United States.[6,7] Because of the rarity of this disease, we lack extensive trials evaluating therapies for WM, current therapies were mainly derived from B-CLL and MM. Things have changed, and now we have novel trials with appreciable numbers of patients with WM.

DEFINITION RELAPSED AND REFRACTORY WALDENSTRÖM'S MACROGLOBULINEMIA

When we face a patient with suspected relapsed or refractory WM (RRWM), we have to follow progressive disease criteria that, according to the 2006 definition, is categorized by >25% increase in serum monoclonal IgM by protein electrophoresis, confirmed in a second measurement, or by the progression of clinically significant findings caused by disease (anemia, thrombocytopenia, leukopenia, or bulky adenopathy/organomegaly) or symptoms (unexplained recurrent fever >38.4°C, drenching night sweats, ≥10% weight loss, hyperviscosity, neuropathy, or symptomatic cryoglobulinemia) attributable to WM.[8]

These criteria were reviewed in 2013[9] due to the increase of complete responses (CR) and very good partial responses (VGPR) reported with the updated therapeutic combinations. As in the International Workshop of WM held in 2002 in Athens,[10] it was again stressed that progression should not necessarily be followed by treatment when this is defined solely based on increasing IgM concentrations. The reappearance of monoclonal IgM protein or recurrence of BM involvement, lymphadenopathy/splenomegaly, or symptoms attributable to active disease defined a relapse from CR. Progression from a partial response (PR) or minor response was defined by >25% increase from the lowest serum IgM level. The development of new signs and symptoms of the disease, including Bing–Neel syndrome and histological transformation, was also considered evidence of disease progression.

CURRENT TREATMENT OPTIONS FOR RELAPSED/REFRACTORY WALDENSTRÖM'S MACROGLOBULINEMIA

Therapy should be initiated in the event of a symptomatic relapse or refractory disease.[11] The treatment depends on different factors that will be reviewed at the end of this review, but no consensus on a preferred regimen exists.[12] A retrospective study with 454 European patients with WM demonstrated that the median progression-free survival (PFS) after first-line therapy was only 29 months. Still, the median OS had not been achieved and the 10-year OS was 69%.[13] This means that second-line and subsequent therapies are very effective in maintaining patients mortality free from WM. In addition, PFS was shorter in patients treated with monotherapy compared to combinations,[13] which reinforce the view that monotherapy should be restricted to a few specific patients, while most should receive combination therapy, especially in second line.[14] This view changed when Bruton tyrosine kinase inhibitors (BTKi) demonstrated high efficacy in monotherapy for patients with RRWM.[15,16]

Table 1
Anti-CD20 combinations with conventional drugs in Waldentröm's macroglobulinemia

Study	N Untreated	Treated	Regimen	ORR	MRR	VGPR + CR	mR	FU	OS	Comments
Souchet et al,[21] 2016	25	57	R 375 mg/m² IV D1, F 40 mg/m² po D1–3, Cy 250 mg/m² po D1–3 ≥2 courses	85%	77%	42%	8%	PFS: 67% at 4 y	90% at 3 y	Grade 3–4 neutropenia, thrombopenia, and anemia of 43%, 13%, and 9%, respectively. Four cases of infection leading to treatment discontinuation
Tedeschi et al,[22] 2012	28	15	R 375 mg/m² IV D1, F 25 mg/m² po D2–4, Cy 250 mg/m² po D2–4 4–6 courses	87%	69%	13%	5%	DR: +14 mo	+20	Neutropenia in 63% Late improvement of responses was observed
Tedeschi et al,[20] 2013	-	40	R 375 mg/m² IV D1, F 25 mg/m² po D2–4, Cy 250 mg/m² po D2–4 4–6 courses	80%	80%	33%	0%	EFS 77 mo	NR	Neutropenia ≥3 (87%), anemia and thrombopenia ≥3 (28%), infections ≥3 (15%)
Laszlo et al,[18] 2010	16	13	R, 375 mg/m² iv D1 Cl, 0.1 mg/kg sc, D1–5 4 courses	90%	79%	24%	10%	-	-	Grade 3–4 neutropenia, 37%; 14% of infections. hCNT1 high expression correlated with the best responses.
Abonour, Buske, Ioakimidis et al[35–37]	47	10	R 375 mg/m² IV, D0 Cy 750 mg/m² IV, D1 Dox 50 mg/m² IV, D1 V 1.4 mg/m² IV (max 2) D1 P 100 mg/m² PO D1–5 6–8 courses, every 21 D	95%	71%	14%	10%	PFS: +20 mo	+36	Neutropenia 3–4 72%. Infections 6%. Alopecia 84%, Nausea/vomiting 36%, mucositis 36%

(continued on next page)

Table 1
(continued)

Study	N Untreated	Treated	Regimen	ORR	MRR	VGPR + CR	mR	FU	OS	Comments
Leblond et al,[19] 2001	-	45	Cy 750 mg/m², D1 Dox 25 mg/m², D1 P 40 mg/m²/day, D1–50 ~6 courses	-	11%	-	-	3 mo	8 mo	>2 Infections (2%), 1 mucositis (4%), and 1 alopecia (5%)
Paludo et al,[25] 2017	-	50	Dex 20 mg/m² po D1, R 375 mg/m² IV D1, Cy 200 mg/m²/day po, D1–5 ~6 courses	87%	68%	4%	19%	FU: 51 mo PFS 32%	74% at 4 y	Grade 3–4 neutropenia, 20%; thrombopenia 7%; infections 3%. Treatment was shortened in 11% due to toxicity.
Arulogun et al,[26] 2020	139	111	R 375 mg/m², D1 Benda, 70–90 mg/m², D1–2 ~6 courses	84%	74%	24%	10%	82% at 2 y	-	Toxicity-related treatment truncation 35%
Treon et al,[27] 2011	-	30	Benda 90 mg/m², D1–2 ± R 375 mg/m², D1 ± (n = 24) O 1000 mg, D1 (n = 6)	83%	66%	17%	17%	13 mo	-	Myelosupression (13%), infection (7%) and hypersensitivity (7%)
Tedeschi et al,[28] 2015	-	71	R 375 mg/m², D1 Benda, 70–90 mg/m², D1–2 ~6 courses	80%	75%	23%	6%	NR at 19 mo	72% at 4 y	Neutropenia (13%), infections (15%), infusion-related reactions (7%). No flare
Paludo et al,[29] 2018	16	44	R 375 mg/m², D1 Benda, 90 mg/m², D1–2 ~6 courses	95%	82%	41%	13%	PFS: 88% at 2 y	-	Neutropenia (11%), infections (5%), thrombocytopenia (2%)

Abbreviations: Benda, bendamustine; Cl, cladribine; CR, complete response; Cy, cyclophosphamide; D, day; Dox, doxorubicin; DR, duration of response; Dx, dexamethasone; F, fludarabine; FU, follow-up; HCNT1, human concentrative nucleoside transporter 1; iv, intravenous; mR, minor response; O, obinutuzumab; ORR, overall response rate; OS, overall survival; P, prednisone; po, per os; PR, partial response; R, rituximab; sc, subcutaneous; TTP, time to tumor progression; V, vincristine; VGPR, very good partial response.

COMBINATIONS WITH CONVENTIONAL CHEMOTHERAPY

Combinations with Nucleoside Analogs

Nucleoside analogs (fludarabine, cladribine) demonstrated high efficacy in treatment-naïve and RR patients,[17–20] especially when combined with cyclophosphamide and rituximab. The overall response rate (ORR), defined as CR + VGPR + PR + minor response (mR), usually exceeds 80%, including a CR rate ~20% (**Table 1**). The median time to response (TTR) is < 3 months and median PFS $\geq$3 years.[18,21,22]

The major disadvantages of purine analogs are the hematologic toxicity and immunosuppressive complications,[11,17,21–23] and a potential increase in Richter's transformation and secondary myelodysplasia (~10%),[23,24] which has relegated the use of these drugs in WM.

Combinations with Alkylating Agents

Alkylating agents (chlorambucil and cyclophosphamide) have been extensively used in monotherapy or combination with steroids.[17] The combination of dexamethasone, rituximab, and cyclophosphamide (DRC) is one of the most popular regimens used as first-line treatment.[13] Moreover, it is also effective in the relapsed population, where it can render an ORR of 87%, with 4% VGPR, 64% PR, and 19% mR.[25]

Bendamustine has been used in both untreated and treated patients with favorable results. The biggest series in the RRWM population included 111 patients treated with rituximab and bendamustine (R-Benda) who were retrospectively evaluated; the major response rate (MRR) and ORR were 74% and 84%, respectively, with a combined CR/VGPR rate of 24%. After a median follow-up of 37 months, only 43% of patients had progressed.[26] Other studies evaluating R-Benda have provided similar results with hematologic adverse events (AEs) as the most relevant safety concerns (see **Table 1**).[27–29] Accordingly, R-Benda is considered an effective treatment but should be used with caution in frail or elderly patients, in whom frequent hospitalizations, infections, and cardiovascular events may be a challenge.[30]

Combinations with Proteasome Inhibitors

Proteasome inhibitors (PIs) have become an important therapeutic strategy in monoclonal gammopathies. Data supporting their use have led to approval for using bortezomib, carfilzomib, and ixazomib in the United States and Europe.[31] These drugs inhibit the ubiquitin-proteasome pathway (UPP), essential for cell survival. UPP inhibition results in toxic protein accumulation for the cells, especially for those specialized in protein production, such as plasma and lymphoplasmacytic cells.

Bortezomib

As a single drug, bortezomib provides 46% to 60% major responses (MRs) in patients with RRWM[32–35] at the conventional dose of 1.3 mg/m^2 (**Table 2**). Bortezomib is generally well tolerated, with usually predictable toxicities, including thrombocytopenia, fatigue, nausea, peripheral neuropathy (PNP), myalgia, non-neutropenic infections, diarrhea, and grade 3–4 constipation in up to 20% of patients, which are manageable with dose reductions or discontinuations (~40% of patients).

Results improved by adding rituximab. A total of 37 patients with RRWM were treated with bortezomib once weekly (1.6 mg/m^2) with rituximab weekly (375 mg/m^2) during courses 1 and 4.[36] The ORR was 81%, including 2 patients (5%) who achieved CR/VGPR and 17 (46%) PR. The most frequent grade 3 toxicity was hematological but manageable, and without relevant PNP. Thanks to these results, bortezomib was successfully moved to first line of therapy.[37–39]

Table 2
Combinations with proteasome inhibitors in Waldenström's macroglobulinemia

First Author Ref	N	Therapy	Cycles	ORR	MRR	VGPR + CR	Outcome	OS	Grade ≥3 Toxicity
Dimopoulos et al,[32] 2005	10	B	4	100%	60%	10%	PFS 40% at 1 y	-	Neutropenia (10%), thrombocytopenia (20%), PNP (20%), fatigue (20%), Ileus (30%)
Chen et al,[104] 2007	27	B	6	78%	44%	-	Median PFS 16 mo	-	Neutropenia (19%), thrombocytopenia (26%), PNP ≥3 (18%), fatigue (11%), myalgia (11%), infections (48%)
Treon et al,[34] 2007	27	B	6	85	48%	0% (CR)	Median TTP 7 mo	-	Neutropenia (14%), thrombocytopenia (7%), PNP (22%), dizziness (11%)
Ghobrial et al,[36] 2010	37	BR	6	88%	66%	8%	Median PFS 16 mo	96% at 1 y	Neutropenia (12%), Thrombocytopenia (8%), Anemia (8%), PNP (0%)
Leblond et al,[35] 2017	34	BD	6	75%	43%	4%	Median PFS 15 mo	84% at 2 y	Thrombocytopenia (35%), anemia (29%), and neutropenia (15%)
Kersten et al,[48] 2022	59	IRD	8	71	85	15	PFS 54% at 2 y	88% at 2 y	Anemia (12%), thrombocytopenia (12%), neutropenia (21%)
Treon et al,[43] 2014	31 (3 R/R)	CaRD	6–14	87%	68%	35%	PFS 65% at 15 mo	-	Dexamethasone-related hyperglycemia (23%), carfilzomib-related hyperlipasemia (16%), and neutropenia (6.5%). PNP irrelevant
Vesole et al,[44] 2018	7	Ca		100%	86%	43%	Median PFS 19 mo	-	Cytopenia, neuropathy

Abbreviations: B, bortezomib; Ca, Carfilzomib; D, dexamethasone; HQR, high-quality responses (CR + VGPR); I, ixazomib; MRR, major response rate; ORR, overall response rate; OS, overall survival; PFS, progression-free survival; PNP, peripheral neuropathy; R, rituximab; WM, Waldentröm's macroglobulinemia.

The combination of everolimus, bortezomib, and rituximab was tested in 46 patients with RRWM.[40] Although the combination produced an ORR of 89% with a MRR of 53%, and the median PFS was 21 months, there were 63% treatment-related toxicities (fatigue, anemia, leucopenia, neutropenia, and/or diarrhea), which have put this regimen behind other better tolerable options.

There is a real-world experience with bortezomib-containing regimens in 32 patients with RRWM, including 10 (30%) who were refractory or intolerant to BTKi.[41] The ORR was 86%: CR 18%, VGPR 18%, PR 44%, and mR 4%. The 2-year OS and PFS was 90% and 76%, respectively. PNP (grade 1–2) occurred in 24% of patients but resulting only in 1 discontinuation. MRR was comparable between previously exposed or not to BTKi (84% vs. 75%, respectively).

Carfilzomib

Carfilzomib is another PI not only tolerable and active in monoclonal gammopathies, but also virtually free of neurotoxicity,[31] although this could be hampered by some cardiovascular problems.[42] The Dana–Farber group examined the combination of carfilzomib, rituximab, and dexamethasone (CaRD) in 31 symptomatic patients with WM, but only 3 of them had been previously treated with chemotherapy.[43] The ORR was 87% (1 CR, 10 VGPR, 10 PR, and 6 mR), and the PFS was 60% at 18 months. Most frequent toxicity was hyperglycemia, present in all patients at any grade (26% grade 3). PNP was notably reduced with respect to BDR (3%, grade 2), whereas cardiopathy, typically associated to carfilzomib, appeared only in 1 patient. There is an experience with CaRD in 7 patients with RR, with an ORR of 86%, 19 months of PFS, and a 14% of PNP/cardiopathy.[44]

Ixazomib

Ixazomib is an oral PI with limited neurotoxicity active and safe in MM.[45] These characteristics and its convenient once weekly oral administration has stimulated the use of ixazomib combined with dexamethasone and rituximab (IRD). This combination is useful in previously untreated patients with symptomatic WM,[46] so it has also been tested in RRWM. The Mayo Clinic presented the preliminary results of ixazomib plus ibrutinib for WM (NCT03506373),[47] in 21 patients: 9 newly diagnosed (ND)WM and 12 RRWM. The ORR was 76%, VGPRs 24%, PR 52%, mR 14%, and SD 10%, with no main differences between NDWM and RRWM. Although most patients developed AEs, very few were of grade 3–4: neutropenia (3 patients) and, anemia, hypertension, hypoxia, peripheral sensory neuropathy, and lung infection in 2 patients each.

The HOVON group carried out a trial in RRWM patients with IRD.[48] A total of 59 patients were enrolled with a median age of 69 years and a median of 2 prior treatments was 2 (range, 1–7). Response and survival were excellent (**Table 3**), and the toxicity was manageable: grade 2–3 cytopenias, grade 1–2 PNP, and grade 2–3 infections, demonstrating that the IRD regimen is efficient and tolerable.

Approved Bruton Tyrosine Kinase Inhibitors

B-cell receptor (BCR) signaling plays a central role in the survival support and growth of malignant B-cells in patients with B-cell lymphoproliferative disorders. This is especially relevant in WM, considering the major role of MYD88 mutation in the pathogenesis of WM. Accordingly, BTK currently represents a potent therapeutic target also in RR disease.[12,49] Its efficacy and use in clinical practice is rapidly changing the management of B-cell malignancies, including WM (see **Table 2**; **Table 4**).

Ibrutinib

Ibrutinib is the first-in-class inhibitor of BTK, displaying a unique targeted mechanism of action by inhibiting downstream signaling after interaction between the mutated

Table 3
Bruton tyrosine kinase inhibitors in Waldenström's macroglobulinemia

Study: 1st Author Ref	N	ORR %	CR + GVPR %	PR%	Median FU Time	Outcomes	Grade ≥3 Toxicity
Ibrutinib							
Treon et al,[15] 2015	63	91	30	49	59 mo	Median PFS: NR. 5-y PFS rate: 54%	Neutropenia 15%, thrombocytopenia 13%, CVE (grade 1–2) 15%, PNP 0%
Trotman et al,[52] 2021	31	87	29	48	58 mo	Median PFS: 39 mo. 60 mo PFS rate: 40%	Neutropenia 10%, thrombocytopenia 3%, CVE (grade 1–2) 16%, PNP 0%
Tam et al,[59] 2020	81	94	20	61	19 mo	Median PFS: NR. 18 mo PFS rate: 82%	Hypertension (11%), atrial fibrillation (4%), neutropenia (8%), anemia (5%), pneumonia (7%)
Ibrutinib + Rituximab							
Dimopoulos et al,[105] 2018	41	93	34	42	50 mo	Median PFS: NR. 54 mo PFS rate: 68%	Hypertension (13%), atrial fibrillation (12%), anemia (11%), and infusion-related reactions (1%)
Zanubrutinib							
Trotman et al,[52] 2021	53	94	51	29	36 mo	Median PFS: NR 36 mo PFS rate; 76.2%	CVE (grade 1–2) 6%, infection 3%
An et al,[58] 2021	43	77	33	37	33 mo	Median PFS: NR 24 mo PFS rate: 60.5%	CVE (grade 1–2) 6%, infection 3%
Tam et al,[59] 2020	83	94	29	49	19 mo	Median PFS: NR 18 mo PFS rate: 86%	Hypertension (6%), atrial fibrillation (0%), neutropenia (20%), anemia (5%), pneumonia (1%)
Acalabrutinib							
Owen et al,[62] 2020	92	95	27	57	63.7 mo	Median PFS: 67.5 mo 66 mo PFS rate: 52%	CVE (grade 1–2) 6%, infection 3%
Tirabrutinib							
Sekiguchi et al,[64] 2022	9	89	33	56	25 mo	Median PFS: NR 24 mo PFS rate: 88.9%	Neutropenia (22%), lymphopenia (19%), and leukopenia (11%)
Orelabrutinib							
Cao et al,[65] 2022	9	89	21.3	60	16 mo	Median PFS NR: 12 mo	Neutropenia (10.6%), leukocytopenia (6.4%), thrombocytopenia (6.4%), and pneumonia (4.3%)

Abbreviations: CVE, cardiovascular events; HQR, high-quality responses (CR + VGPR); NR, not reached; ORR, overall response rate; PFS, progression-free survival; PNP, peripheral neuropathy; PR, partial response; WM, Waldentröm macroglobulinemia.

Table 4
Selected adverse events reported in clinical trials with BTK inhibitors in patients with Waldenström's macroglobulinemia

	Ibrutinib Treon et al,[15] 2015	Ibrutinib Tam et al,[59] 2020	Ibrutinib R Buske et al,[54] 2020	Zanubrutinib Trotman et al,[52] 2021	Zanubrutinib Tam et al,[59] 2020	Acalabrutinib Owen et al,[62] 2020	Tirabrutinib Seghiguki et al,[64] 2022	Orelabrutinib Cao et al,[65] 2022
FU	59 mo	44 mo	50 mo	36 mo	44 mo	63.7 mo	24.8 mo	16.4 mo
AE leading to drug discontinuation %	7.9	20.4	11	13	8.9	16	0	6.4
AE leading to dose reduction %	19	26.5	22.6	NR	15.8	NR	NR	NR
Hematological toxicity								
Neutropenia grade 3/4%	15.8	10.2	13	15.6	23.8	17	44	10.6
Anemia grade 3/4%	1.6	6.1	12	-	11.9	6	0	0
Thrombocytopenia grade 3/4%	11.1	6.1	1	9.1	10.9	NR	0	6.5
Infection grade 3/4%	6.3	27.6	29	27.3	21.8	33	0	8.5
Pneumonia grade 3/4%	3.1	10.2	11	3.9	1	9	0	4.3
Atrial fibrillation any grade %	12.7	23.5	19	-	7.9	12	11	0
Hypertension grade 3/4%	0	20.4	15	3.9	8.9	4	0	0
Bleeding grade 3/4%	NR	10.2	7	3.8	8.9	7	0	2.1
Diarrhea grade 3/4%	0	2	NR	2.6	3	NR	0	0

Abbreviations: AE, adverse event; BTK, Bruton tyrosine kinase; NR, not reached; WM, Waldentröm macroglobulinemia.

MYD88 protein and BTK. It was approved by the FDA in 2015 for symptomatic WM[50] based on the results of an investigator-initiated multicenter phase II study in 63 symptomatic previously treated patients in whom ibrutinib exerted a rapid increase in hemoglobin levels and rapid decreases in serum IgM.[15] At the extended follow-up of 59 months, in a population of heavily pretreated patients (median 2 prior lines, 40% refractory), ibrutinib monotherapy induced an ORR of 91%, an MRR of 71%, and 30% VGPR. Importantly, the 5-year PFS rate was 54%. Treatment with 3 or more versus 1 to 2 prior lines of therapy significantly impacted PFS duration (5-year PFS rate, 38% vs. 68%; $P = .01$), suggesting the preferred early use of ibrutinib in case of progression in BTKi-naïve patients.[51] $CXCR4^{mut}$ cases, compared with $CXCR4^{WT}$, had a lower MRR (68% vs. 97%), and VGPR (47% vs. 9%), as well as longer median time to MRR (4.7 vs. 1.8 months). No MRs were observed in the 4 $MYD88^{WT}$ patients. PFS was not reached in patients with $MYD88^{mut}/CXCR4^{WT}$, 4.5 years for $MYD88^{mut}/CXCR4^{mut}$, and 4 months for $MYD88^{WT}$ patients.

Ibrutinib is effective even in the setting of rituximab refractory patients. In the arm C of the phase III iNNOVATE trial, the BTKi given as a single agent in 31 rituximab refractory and heavily pretreated patients attained a high ORR (87%) including 29% VGPR, with a median PFS of 39 months.[16] As in the pivotal trial, PFS was better for $MYD88^{mut}/CXCR4^{WT}$ versus 18 months in $MYD88^{mut}/CXCR4^{mut}$.[52]

In the multicenter iNNOVATE study,[53,54] patients with WM, mostly RR, were randomized to receive ibrutinib in combination with rituximab (IR) versus placebo-rituximab. IR demonstrated robust responses close to 80% or above that were consistent across all $MYD88$ and $CXCR4$ genotype subsets, suggesting that the combination can potentially overcome the relatively low responses seen with ibrutinib single-agent treatment in unfavorable genotypes. In RRWM, the 54-month PFS rate was 68% with IR versus 20% with placebo-rituximab and the PFS benefit was seen regardless of $MYD88$ and $CXCR4$ mutation status.

Some studies have evaluated ibrutinib in common clinical practice. In a series of 54 patients with RRWM,[55] the response raters (ORR and MRR) were consistent with those reported in clinical trials (ORR 89% with 78% MRR) and the discontinuation rate (21%).[15] There is also a comparison between patients treated with ibrutinib monotherapy on and off clinical trials.[56] The rate and depth of responses of 157 patients treated in common practice were comparable to that of patients on clinical trials. No significant difference was observed in the 4-year PFS of 72% versus 63% between ON and OFF trial patients, respectively ($P = .14$).

Zanubrutinib

Zanubrutinib was developed to maximize BTK inhibition and avoid off-target effects. In the first trial (phase I/II) evaluating the role of zanubrutinib in WM, there were 53 patients with RRWM.[57] ORR after 36 months of follow-up was high (94%), and MR was seen in 80% patients with RR with a median time to response of 2.8 months. A total of 39% achieved a VGPR at 12 months, and 51% at 24 months. Similar results with a favorable VGPR or better (33%) and response benefit independent from genotype were observed in the phase II Chinese study after a median follow-up of 33 months.[58]

The ASPEN trial is a head-to-head study comparing ibrutinib with zanubrutinib with the primary endpoint of achieving better CRs plus VGPRs in patients receiving the new BTKi.[59] $MYD88^{MUT}$ patients were randomized to receive 1 of the 2 inhibitors, whereas those with $MYD88^{WT}$ received directly zanubrutinib.[53] Most patients enrolled in cohort 1 had RR disease. The primary objective was not met (28% with zanubrutinib vs. 19% with ibrutinib $P = .09$). There was no difference in ORR with zanubrutinib compared to ibrutinib (94% vs. 93%, respectively), or in MRR (77% vs. 78%) or 18 months PFS (84% vs. 85%). Median time to achieve at least a VGPR was shorter for zanubrutinib (7 months) compared to ibrutinib (17 months).[60] PFS rate at 42 months was not significantly different. A longer follow-up has demonstrated that patients carrying $CXCR4^{MUT}$ achieved a deeper response with zanubrutinib (21% vs. 10%), faster responses, and better PFS (42 months PFS rate: 73% vs. 42%).

In patients without $MYD88$ mutation of the cohort 2 of the ASPEN trial, zanubrutinib led to a 65% MRR, with 31% VGPRs and CRs. At 42 months, PFS was 52%. In 2021, zanubrutinib was approved by the FDA and EMA for patients with WM.[53,60]

A phase II expanded access study with zanubrutinib enrolled 50 patients in the United States,[61] and 33 patients with RRWM treated with a median of 2 prior lines. The median duration exposure was 10 months, with 90% of patients achieving a response with a high rate of VGPR (43%). The favorable toxicity profile was confirmed.

Nonapproved Covalent Bruton Tyrosine Kinase Inhibitors

Acalabrutinib
The second-generation BTKi acalabrutinib (ACP-196) was developed to be more potent and selective than ibrutinib. In WM it was evaluated in monotherapy in a series of 108 patients, 92 of them were RRWM.[62,63] After 64 months of median drug exposure, ORR and MRR were 95% and 84%, respectively, with 4% of patients reaching a CR and 23% a VGPR according to the sixth IWWM response criteria. ORR was consistent across prespecified subgroups (age, IgM level, prior lines of therapy, ECOG). In this study, we do not have data on the impact of genotype as the $CXCR4$ mutational status was not analyzed. The median duration of response and PFS was reached at 64.7 and 67.5 months, respectively. Up to now, acalabrutinib has not been approved by the regulatory agencies and no direct comparison of acalabrutinib with the other BTKi is available in patients with WM.

Tirabrutinib
Tirabrutinib was evaluated in 27 patients in a phase II monotherapy study at a daily dose of 480 mg in both treatment naïve and RRWM. Tirabrutinib exerted high response rates (ORR 96%) with rates of MRR similar in both patients with TN and R/R (89% in both), time to overall and MR was of 1 and 2 months, respectively. Of the 9, 3 patients with RR reached a good quality of response. At the 2-year follow-up, only 2 patients had discontinued treatment due to disease progression.[64] In August 2020, tirabrutinib was approved in Japan for patients with TN or R/R WM and LPL.

Orelabrutinib
Orelabrutinib is a novel, small molecule, selective irreversible BTKi investigated in a multicenter phase II trial in 47 patients with R/R. After a median time to response of 1.9 months, 89% of patients reached a response, with 21% achieving at least a VGPR. The follow-up of the study is still short. The estimated 12-month PFS is 89%.[65]

Noncovalent Bruton tyrosine kinase inhibitors
Pirtobrutinib. Pirtobrutinib is a highly selective, noncovalent (reversible) BTKi with promising efficacy in patients with RR B-cell malignancies.[66] The BRUIN study included 78 RRWM with a median age of 68 years and a median of 3 prior therapies.[67] A total of 85% patients had received chemoimmunotherapy alone, and 64% had received a BTKi (n = 61). Among the latter, 66% had discontinued prior BTKi due to disease progression. The MRR was 68%, including 24% VGPRs and 44% PRs. With a median follow-up of 8 months, the 6-month estimated duration of response (DoR) rate was 86%. In the BTKi-pretreated subset, the 6-month DoR was 83%.

Considering all B-cell malignancies treated with pirtobrutinib (n = 725), the most frequent AEs were fatigue (26%), diarrhea (22%), and contusion (19%). Neutropenia grade ≥3 was present in 20%, hypertension in 3%, hemorrhage in 2%, and atrial fibrillation/flutter in 1%. Overall, 2% of patients discontinued due to a treatment-related AE.[67]

Nemtabrutinib. Nemtabrutinib (MK-1026, formerly ARQ-531) is a noncovalent, potent inhibitor of both wild-type and ibrutinib-resistant C481S-mutated BTK,[68] the most common mechanism of resistance to covalent BTKis.[69] This drug was tested in 112 heavily pretreated patients with RR B-cell malignancies,[70] including 6 patients with WM. Responses were promising and toxicity manageable. No data are yet available for WM, but responses are possible, and data will be available from the NCT03162536 ongoing trial.

Bruton Tyrosine Kinase Inhibitors Adverse Events

BTKi treatment requires continuous administration for an indefinite course. Although treatment with BTKi is generally well tolerated and many early secondary effects usually decrease over time, prolonged drug exposure may translate into a progressively increased rate of AE. A major concern with continuous treatment is the development of AEs leading to intolerance and definitive treatment discontinuation, which translates into a poor prognosis. Ibrutinib's abrupt discontinuations to manage AE may be associated with a quick increase of IgM and potential withdrawal symptoms such as fever, body aches, headache, and arthralgias.[71]

Table 4 reports the definitive discontinuations and dosage reduction rates due to AE seen in large clinical trials. It is difficult to compare the tolerability of the BTKi as studies have different observation periods and characteristics of enrolled patients. The only study allowing a direct head-to-head comparison of AEs with ibrutinib and zanubrutinib is the ASPEN randomized trial.

Ibrutinib exerts the highest off-target effects. Patients often see atrial fibrillation, hypertension, hemorrhages, diarrhea, arthralgia, and rash, although most episodes are limited to grade 1–2.[72] Ventricular arrhythmias are uncommon, but they are the most worrisome toxicity of ibrutinib, and have also been reported with acalabrutinib.[73] Risk factors associated with atrial fibrillation are advanced age, prior history of cardiopathies, and hypertension, which the BTKi may induce. Next-generation BTKi have minimized off-target toxicities, so they have less AEs and better tolerability. Although atrial fibrillation and hypertension have also been reported with acalabrutinib and zanubrutinib, these AEs were more frequent with ibrutinib.[62,74]

Other frequent grade ≥3 AE with BTKis are cytopenias, specifically neutropenia (range 10%–24%). Grade 3–4 infections are highly interesting in WM, and they are frequent, particularly during the early treatment period, especially upper respiratory tract infections and pneumonia.[51,62,74]

The limited number of patients treated with tirabrutinib and orelabrutinib does not allow drawing any conclusion, although atrial fibrillation and hypertension have been observed in a low frequency.[64,65]

The direct comparison of zanubrutinib with ibrutinib showed that the former was better tolerated and associated with a lower risk of AEs leading to dose reductions (16% vs. 27%), treatment discontinuation (9% vs. 20%), or death (3% vs. 5%). Several AEs were statistically more frequent with ibrutinib than with zanubrutinib, including atrial fibrillation, hypertension, diarrhea, peripheral edema, muscle spasms, and pneumonia ($P < .05$ for all comparisons). In contrast, neutropenia occurred more frequently with zanubrutinib ($P < .05$), although did not translate into more infections.[59]

Stem Cell Transplant

Stem cell transplantation (SCT) has been shown to produce durable responses with a treatment-related mortality rate of 3.8%, although virtually all data came from retrospective studies.[75] Good outcomes were seen with high-dose treatment; 5-year PFS and OS rates were 40% and 69%, respectively.[76] In total, 22% of patients achieved a CR after ASCT. Data on allogeneic SCT are also derived from retrospective studies only. A retrospective series of 144 patients with WM demonstrated an OS of 74% after 1 year and 52% after 5 years, with PFS of 68% and 46%, respectively. The 1- and 5-year nonrelapse mortality was 15% and 30%, respectively.[77] SCT is less recommended in WM at present because of its high toxicity and the existence of more tolerable therapies.

OTHER EMERGING TREATMENTS
BCL2 Inhibitors

Venetoclax

BCL2 is an apoptosis inhibitor overexpressed in WM.[78] Venetoclax is a selective BCL2 inhibitor that is very effective in several hematological malignancies. In a phase II trial, 32 patients with RRWM received 200 to 800 mg venetoclax daily for 2 years, including 16 previously exposed to BTKis. The median FU was 33 months, and ORR and MRR were 84 and 81%, respectively. The median PFS was 30 months. MRR was lower in refractory versus relapsed patients (50% vs. 95%; $P = .007$). Neutropenia was the only occurring grade ≥ 3 AE (45%), including 1 episode of febrile neutropenia. No tumor lysis syndrome was observed, except one case with abnormal laboratory findings. Grade 2 AEs were seen in most patients (94%), mostly anemia, lymphopenia, and neutropenia. Temporary drug hold occurred in 14 patients, usually due to neutropenia, infections, or diarrhea. A phase II trial assessing the combination of venetoclax with ibrutinib in NDWM was done, with interesting results, but with an excess of ventricular arrhythmia, including 2 sudden deaths, which caused a full clinical hold on this trial.[79]

Phosphatidylinositol 3-Kinase Inhibitors

Phosphatidylinositol 3-kinase inhibitors have provided good results in indolent B-cell lymphoproliferative disorders,[80] so they are interesting for WM. Idelalisib, one of the most popular ones, combined with obinutuzumab demonstrated an ORR of 71% and a median PFS of 25 months,.[81] Still, no further development has been pursued due to excess toxicity.[81,82]

Antibodies

Anti-CXCR4 monoclonal antibodies

CXCR4 mutations are present in 30% to 40% of patients with WM.[1] They can impact the clinical and biological behavior of patient with WM.[83] Thus, targeting CXCR4 in WM has been assessed in clinical trials. Ulocuplumab is a CXCR4 antagonist evaluated with ibrutinib in 13 patients with WM (4 RR) in whom the CXCR4 had been demonstrated.[84] This combination resulted in an MRR of 100% with a predicted 2-year PFS of 90%, but the drug development has been stopped. Another CXCR4 antagonist, mavorixafor, has been tested with ibrutinib in 9 patients with WM with $MYD88$ and $CXCR4^{WHIM}$, providing a 100% ORR with only 9 AEs (79% grade 1) attributed to mavorixafor, and just two grade 2 AEs leading to discontinuation.[85]

Anti-PD1 antibodies

PD-1 has been implicated in T-cell regulatory function in the WM microenvironment.[86] Actually, PD-1 is expressed on B-cells in WM, promoting malignant cell viability and proliferation.[87] There is, therefore, a rationale to investigate the efficacy of PD-1 blockade in WM.

The UK group developed the PEMBROWM trial to determine the safety, tolerability, and efficacy of pembrolizumab in combination with rituximab in RRWM previously exposed to covalent BTKis (NCT03630042).[88] A total of 17 patients had been initially registered, with median age of 70 years, and the majority (n = 15) having received a BTKi as the last therapy. With a median follow-up of 15 months, the ORR after 24 weeks was 47%, with 6% attaining VGPR, 18% PR, 18% mR, and 6% with an unavailable response but with evidence of mR at week 12. The median PFS was 13 months, and the median OS was not reached. There were 3 discontinuations due to AE: immune thrombocytopenia (1), and infection (2, including one COVID-19 infection), but most AEs were grade 1–2. Accordingly, pembrolizumab demonstrated safety, tolerability, and potential efficacy combined with rituximab, which requires future trials to demonstrate its real efficacy in WM.

There is a small experience with atezolizumab (anti-PD-L1) in combination with anti-CD20 in patients with RRMCL (n = 30), WM (n = 4), or MZL (n = 21).[89] Although results were encouraging in MCL and MZL, no responses were seen in WM, so this strategy should be changed for the future.

Tislelizumab combined with zanubrutinib has been tested in RR B-cell malignancies (NCT02795182).[90] However, 2 patients with WM developed a direct antiglobulin test negative severe hemolytic anemia,[91] so WM was removed from the trial.

Anti-CD38

Expression of CD38, a marker of plasmacytoid differentiation, can be seen by immunohistochemistry in a subset of patients with WM.[92] Daratumumab, an anti-CD38 monoclonal antibody highly active in CD38+ plasma cell dyscrasias,[93] was tested in a phase 2 trial as monotherapy in 13 patients with RRWM. The trial yielded disappointing results, with an ORR of 23%, MRR of 15%, and median PFS of 2 months,[94] justified by the low intensity of CD38 expression in the surface of WM cells by flow cytometry.[95] Additional trials are ongoing, such as the NCT03679624 evaluating daratumumab combined with ibrutinib.

Anti-CD19

WM cells are positive for CD19 so this antigen could be the target for another directed therapy. Loncastuximab tesirine (ADCT-402) is an antibody-drug conjugate comprising anti-CD19 conjugated to a pyrrolobenzodiazepine dimer toxin. There is an experience with this compound in RR B-cell NHL (NCT02669017).[96] The trial demonstrated efficacy and tolerability, but only 1 patient with WM was recruited. A new trial with loncastuximab tesirine is under development led by the Boston group (NCT05190705).

T-cell Therapies

Chimeric antigen receptor (CAR) T-cell therapy is being introduced within the spectrum of all B-disorders.[97] CAR T therapy is highly efficacious in diffuse large B-cell lymphoma and acute lymphoblastic leukemia, and it is being accepted for mantle cell lymphoma[98] and CLL.[99] However, the experience is limited in WM. Only 3 very heavily treated patients with WM have been treated with CAR-T therapy.[100] This experience demonstrated that treatment was tolerated, and toxicities were consistent with those seen for CAR-T in other diseases. All 3 patients attained at least a clinical response, including 1 minimal residual disease-negative CR. A prospective trial for rare B-cell lymphoproliferative disorders will include around 60 patients with RRWM (NCT05537766).

Bispecific antibodies, another T-cell targeted immune therapy, are active in indolent NHLs, including WM.[101] In a phase I trial with a CD20xCD3 bispecific antibody in relapsed/refractory B-NHL including 3 RRWM, the most commonly reported grade 3 AEs were anemia, lymphopenia, infections, and neutropenia. Although the stimulating results in other diseases make bispecific antibodies a very attractive option in WM, they need more available data, making exploring them in prospective clinical trials urgent.

Other Therapies

Iopofosine I[131] (CLR 131) is a targeted radiotherapeutic that has demonstrated efficacy in multiple myeloma,[102] although some efficacy has also been seen in WM (unpublished data). Accordingly, a phase II trial has been started to evaluate iopofosine in RRWM (NCT02952508).

WHICH THERAPY SHOULD WE CHOOSE?

Not all patients have to be treated. Pure biochemical relapses should not be treated, and a close monitorization should be used. If we face a patient with RRWM that requires treatment, the type of therapy must be individualized. Type of treatment should strictly depend on host and disease-related factors and prior therapy (**Fig. 1**).[12,49] The median response duration for the most frequent first-line therapies is 3, 5, and 6 years, for CDR, BDR, and Benda-R, respectively.[12,49] Accordingly, a longer response duration should suggest repeating the prior regimen. The most common limit used for such a decision is usually 3 years based on expert opinion,[49] but it will always depend on the treating hematologist. If the decision is the use of a different therapy, certain treatment attributes should be considered in the selection of salvage treatment such as duration (fixed duration vs. ongoing), potential toxicity, and the type of prior therapies, to select a different mechanism of action. Accordingly, if the patient has received chemoimmunotherapy as the first-line therapy, selecting a BTKi is the best option. If the first-line therapy was a BTKi, for the second line, we should select any of the combos with chemoimmunotherapy (see **Fig. 1**). In addition, the patient's age, comorbidities, and patient and physician preferences could further aid in selecting the best treatment

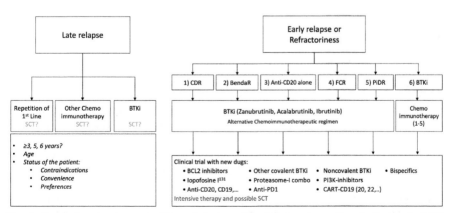

Fig. 1. Strategies at relapse: options of therapy. BendaR, bendamustine & rituximab; BTKi, Bruton tyrosine kinase inhibitor; CDR, cyclophosphamide, dexamethasone & rituximab; FCR, fludarabine, cyclophosphamide, rituximab; PiDR, proteasome inhibitor, dexamethasone and rituximab; RTX, rituximab; SCT, stem cell transplantation.

for a specific patient. For instance, patients with WM prefer fixed-duration treatment with the highest efficacy and the lowest risk of secondary malignancy.[103] Moreover, if the patient is young enough and does not harbor specific comorbidities, we must consider using an SCT, which always promises deep and long-term remissions.[75]

When selecting the therapy for a patient with WM, including salvage therapy, we recommend participating in clinical trials when possible. It could be the only possibility to access new drugs, which is especially relevant for patients who have already received chemoimmunotherapy and covalent BTKis.

CLINICS CARE POINTS

- If long-term PFS was achieved with initial therapy, the regimen can be repeated.
- If toxicity was a concern during first-line therapy, another approach should be made.
- If repeat initial therapy is not the option for your RRWM patient, after chemoimmunotherapy, use a BTK inhibitor; after BTKi failure, use chemoimmunotherapy.
- Pay attention to heart rate, blood pressure, bleeding, and absolute neutrophil counts when using BTK inhibitors.
- If your patient develops toxicity under BTKi therapy, stop for a short period until it is resolved and reinitiate at a lower dose.
- Pay attention to therapy interruptions during BTKi therapy; a relevant increase in the monoclonal protein can be seen (rebound phenomenon).

DISCLOSURE

No potential conflict of interest was reported by the author(s).

FUNDING

RGS received research funding and/or consulting fees from Novartis, Gilead, Astellas, Janssen, Amgen, Takeda, Janssen, Incyte, Astellas, BeiGene, AstraZeneca, Pfizer, and Pharmacyclics. AT declares being on the Advisory Board and Speaker Bureau for Janssen SPA, AbbVie, Astrazeneca, and Beigene.

CONFLICTS OF INTEREST

The authors declare that they have no potential conflicts of interest.

REFERENCES

1. Dogliotti I, Jiménez C, Varettoni M, et al. Diagnostics in Waldenström's macro-globulinemia: a consensus statement of the European Consortium for Waldenström's Macroglobulinemia. Leukemia 2022;37:388–95.
2. Campo E, Jaffe ES, Cook JR, et al. The international consensus classification of mature lymphoid neoplasms: a report from the clinical advisory committee. Blood; 2022.
3. Alaggio R, Amador C, Anagnostopoulos I, et al. The 5th edition of the World health organization classification of haematolymphoid tumours: lymphoid neoplasms. Leukemia 2022;36(7):1720–48.
4. Treon SP, Xu L, Yang G, et al. MYD88 L265P somatic mutation in waldenström's macroglobulinemia. N Engl J Med 2012;367(9):826–33.

5. Jimenez C, Sebastian E, Chillon M, et al. MYD88 L265P is a marker highly characteristic of, but not restricted to, Waldenstrom's macroglobulinemia. Leukemia 2013;27(8):1722–8.

6. Castillo JJ, Olszewski AJ, Kanan S, et al. Survival outcomes of secondary cancers in patients with Waldenström macroglobulinemia: an analysis of the SEER database. Am J Hematol 2015;90(8):696–701.

7. Garcia-Sanz R, Montoto S, Torrequebrada A, et al. Waldenstrom macroglobulinaemia: presenting features and outcome in a series with 217 cases. Br J Haematol 2001;115(3):575–82.

8. Kimby E, Treon SP, Anagnostopoulos A, et al. Update on recommendations for assessing response from the third international workshop on waldenstrom's macroglobulinemia. Clin Lymphoma Myeloma 2006;6(5):380–3.

9. Owen R, Kyle R, Stone M, et al. Response assessment in Waldenstrom macroglobulinaemia: update from the VIth International Workshop. Br J Haematol 2013;160(2):171–6.

10. Weber D, Treon SP, Emmanouilides C, et al. Uniform response criteria in Waldenstrom's macroglobulinemia: consensus panel recommendations from the Second International Workshop on Waldenstrom's Macroglobulinemia. Semin Oncol 2003;30(2):127–31.

11. Leblond V, Kastritis E, Advani R, et al. Treatment recommendations from the Eighth International Workshop on Waldenström's Macroglobulinemia. Blood 2016;128(10):1321–8.

12. Castillo JJ, Advani RH, Branagan AR, et al. Consensus treatment recommendations from the tenth International Workshop for Waldenström Macroglobulinaemia. Lancet Haematol 2020;7(11):e827–37.

13. Buske C, Sadullah S, Kastritis E, et al. Treatment and outcome patterns in European patients with Waldenström's macroglobulinaemia: a large, observational, retrospective chart review. Lancet Haematol 2018;5(7):e299–309.

14. Dimopoulos M, Kastritis E, Owen R, et al. Treatment recommendations for patients with Waldenstrom macroglobulinemia (WM) and related disorders: IWWM-7 consensus. Blood 2014;124(9):1404–11.

15. Treon SP, Tripsas CK, Meid K, et al. Ibrutinib in previously treated Waldenström's macroglobulinemia. N Engl J Med 2015;372(15):1430–40.

16. Dimopoulos MA, Trotman J, Tedeschi A, et al. Ibrutinib for patients with rituximab-refractory Waldenström's macroglobulinaemia (iNNOVATE): an open-label substudy of an international, multicentre, phase 3 trial. Lancet Oncol 2017;18(2):241–50.

17. Garcia-Sanz R, Ocio EM. Novel treatment regimens for Waldenstrom's macroglobulinemia. Expert Rev Hematol 2010;3(3):339–50.

18. Laszlo D, Andreola G, Rigacci L, et al. Rituximab and subcutaneous 2-chloro-2'-deoxyadenosine combination treatment for patients with Waldenstrom macroglobulinemia: clinical and biologic results of a phase II multicenter study. J Clin Oncol 2010;28(13):2233–8.

19. Leblond V, Lévy V, Maloisel F, et al. Multicenter, randomized comparative trial of fludarabine and the combination of cyclophosphamide-doxorubicin-prednisone in 92 patients with Waldenström macroglobulinemia in first relapse or with primary refractory disease. Blood 2001;98(9):2640–4.

20. Tedeschi A, Ricci F, Goldaniga MC, et al. Fludarabine, cyclophosphamide, and rituximab in salvage therapy of Waldenström's macroglobulinemia. Clin Lymphoma Myeloma Leuk 2013;13(2):231–4.

21. Souchet L, Levy V, Ouzegdouh M, et al. Efficacy and long-term toxicity of the rituximab-fludarabine-cyclophosphamide combination therapy in Waldenstrom's macroglobulinemia. Am J Hematol 2016;91(8):782–6.

22. Tedeschi A, Benevolo G, Varettoni M, et al. Fludarabine plus cyclophosphamide and rituximab in Waldenstrom macroglobulinemia: an effective but myelosuppressive regimen to be offered to patients with advanced disease. Cancer 2012;118(2):434–43.

23. Leleu X, Soumerai J, Roccaro A, et al. Increased incidence of transformation and myelodysplasia/acute leukemia in patients with waldenstrom macroglobulinemia treated with nucleoside analogs. J Clin Oncol 2009;27(2):250–5.

24. Leblond V, Tamburini J, Levy V, et al. Incidence of disease transformation and development of MDS/AML in 165 patients with waldenstrom's macroglobulinemia (WM) treated with fludarabine (F)-based regimen in three studies (French Cooperative Group on CLL/WM). ASH Annual Meeting Abstracts 2007;110(11): 1291.

25. Paludo J, Abeykoon JP, Kumar S, et al. Dexamethasone, rituximab and cyclophosphamide for relapsed and/or refractory and treatment-naïve patients with Waldenstrom macroglobulinemia. Br J Haematol 2017;179(1):98–105.

26. Arulogun S, Brian D, Goradia H, et al. Bendamustine Plus Rituximab for the Treatment of Waldenström Macroglobulinaemia: Patient Outcomes and Impact of Bendamustine Dosing. Blood 2020;136(Supl.1):2.

27. Treon SP, Hanzis C, Tripsas C, et al. Bendamustine therapy in patients with relapsed or refractory Waldenström's macroglobulinemia. Clin Lymphoma Myeloma Leuk 2011;11(1):133–5.

28. Tedeschi A, Picardi P, Ferrero S, et al. Bendamustine and rituximab combination is safe and effective as salvage regimen in Waldenström macroglobulinemia. Leuk Lymphoma 2015;56(9):2637–42.

29. Paludo J, Abeykoon JP, Shreders A, et al. Bendamustine and rituximab (BR) versus dexamethasone, rituximab, and cyclophosphamide (DRC) in patients with Waldenström macroglobulinemia. Ann Hematol 2018;97(8):1417–25.

30. Olszewski AJ, Butera JN, Reagan JL, et al. Outcomes of bendamustine- or cyclophosphamide-based first-line chemotherapy in older patients with indolent B-cell lymphoma. Am J Hematol 2020;95(4):354–61.

31. Manasanch EE, Orlowski RZ. Proteasome inhibitors in cancer therapy. Nat Rev Clin Oncol 2017;14(7):417–33.

32. Dimopoulos MA, Anagnostopoulos A, Kyrtsonis MC, et al. Treatment of relapsed or refractory Waldenstrom's macroglobulinemia with bortezomib. Haematologica 2005;90(12):1655–8.

33. Strauss SJ, Maharaj L, Hoare S, et al. Bortezomib therapy in patients with relapsed or refractory lymphoma: potential correlation of in vitro sensitivity and tumor necrosis factor alpha response with clinical activity. J Clin Oncol 2006;24(13):2105–12.

34. Treon SP, Hunter ZR, Matous J, et al. Multicenter clinical trial of bortezomib in relapsed/refractory Waldenstrom's macroglobulinemia: results of WMCTG Trial 03-248. Clin Cancer Res 2007;13(11):3320–5.

35. Leblond V, Morel P, Dilhuidy MS, et al. A phase II Bayesian sequential clinical trial in advanced Waldenström macroglobulinemia patients treated with bortezomib: interest of addition of dexamethasone. Leuk Lymphoma 2017;58(11): 2615–23.

36. Ghobrial IM, Hong F, Padmanabhan S, et al. Phase II trial of weekly bortezomib in combination with rituximab in relapsed or relapsed and refractory Waldenstrom macroglobulinemia. J Clin Oncol 2010;28(8):1422–8.

37. Treon SP, Ioakimidis L, Soumerai JD, et al. Primary therapy of waldenstrom macroglobulinemia with bortezomib, dexamethasone, and rituximab: WMCTG clinical trial 05-180. J Clin Oncol 2009;27(23):3830–5.

38. Dimopoulos MA, Garcia-Sanz R, Gavriatopoulou M, et al. Primary therapy of Waldenstrom macroglobulinemia (WM) with weekly bortezomib, low-dose dexamethasone, and rituximab (BDR): long-term results of a phase 2 study of the European Myeloma Network (EMN). Blood 2013;122(19):3276–82.

39. Gavriatopoulou M, Garcia-Sanz R, Kastritis E, et al. BDR in newly diagnosed patients with WM: final analysis of a phase 2 study after a minimum follow-up of 6 years. Blood 2017;129(4):456–9.

40. Ghobrial IM, Redd R, Armand P, et al. Phase I/II trial of everolimus in combination with bortezomib and rituximab (RVR) in relapsed/refractory Waldenstrom macroglobulinemia. Leukemia 2015;29(12):2338–46.

41. Khwaja J, Uppal E, Baker R, et al. Bortezomib-based therapy is effective and well tolerated in frontline and multiply pre-treated Waldenström macroglobulinaemia including BTKi failures: a real-world analysis. EJHaem 2022;3(4):1330–4.

42. Dimopoulos MA, Moreau P, Palumbo A, et al. Carfilzomib and dexamethasone versus bortezomib and dexamethasone for patients with relapsed or refractory multiple myeloma (ENDEAVOR): a randomised, phase 3, open-label, multicentre study. Lancet Oncol 2016;17(1):27–38.

43. Treon SP, Tripsas CK, Meid K, et al. Carfilzomib, rituximab, and dexamethasone (CaRD) treatment offers a neuropathy-sparing approach for treating Waldenstrom's macroglobulinemia. Blood 2014;124(4):503–10.

44. Vesole DH, Richter J, Biran N, et al. Carfilzomib as salvage therapy in Waldenstrom macroglobulinemia: a case series. Leuk Lymphoma 2018;59(1):259–61.

45. Moreau P, Masszi T, Grzasko N, et al. Oral ixazomib, lenalidomide, and dexamethasone for multiple myeloma. N Engl J Med 2016;374(17):1621–34.

46. Castillo JJ, Meid K, Gustine J, et al. Prospective phase II Study of ixazomib, dexamethasone and rituximab in previously untreated patients with waldenström macroglobulinemia. Blood 2017;130(Suppl 1):1487.

47. Ailawadhi S, Parrondo RD, Laplant B, et al. Phase II study of ibrutinib in combination with ixazomib in patients with waldenström macroglobulinemia (WM). Blood 2022;140(Supplement 1):9331–2.

48. Kersten MJ, Amaador K, Minnema MC, et al. Combining ixazomib with subcutaneous rituximab and dexamethasone in relapsed or refractory waldenström's macroglobulinemia: final analysis of the phase I/II HOVON124/ECWM-R2 study. J Clin Oncol 2022;40(1):40–51.

49. Kastritis E, Leblond V, Dimopoulos MA, et al. Waldenström's macroglobulinaemia: ESMO clinical practice guidelines for diagnosis, treatment and follow-up. Ann Oncol 2019;30(5):860–2.

50. Raedler LA. Imbruvica (Ibrutinib): first drug approved for the treatment of patients with waldenström's macroglobulinemia. Am Health Drug Benefits 2016; 9(Spec Feature):89–92.

51. Treon SP, Meid K, Gustine J, et al. Long-term follow-up of ibrutinib monotherapy in symptomatic, previously treated patients with waldenström macroglobulinemia. J Clin Oncol 2021;39(6):565–75.

52. Trotman J, Buske C, Tedeschi A, et al. Single-agent ibrutinib for rituximab-refractory waldenström macroglobulinemia: final analysis of the substudy of the phase III iNNOVATE ™ trial. Clin Cancer Res 2021;27(21):5793–800.

53. Dimopoulos M, Sanz RG, Lee HP, et al. Zanubrutinib for the treatment of MYD88 wild-type Waldenström macroglobulinemia: a substudy of the phase 3 ASPEN trial. Blood Adv 2020;4(23):6009–18.

54. Buske C, Tedeschi A, Trotman J, et al. Five-year follow-up of ibrutinib plus rituximab vs placebo plus rituximab for waldenstrom's macroglobulinemia: final analysis from the randomized phase 3 iNNOVATE (TM) study. Blood 2020; 136(Supplement 1):24–6.

55. Abeykoon JP, Zanwar S, Ansell SM, et al. Ibrutinib monotherapy outside of clinical trial setting in Waldenström macroglobulinaemia: practice patterns, toxicities and outcomes. Br J Haematol 2020;188(3):394–403.

56. Castillo JJ, Sarosiek SR, Gustine JN, et al. Response and survival predictors in a cohort of 319 patients with Waldenström macroglobulinemia treated with ibrutinib monotherapy. Blood Adv 2022;6(3):1015–24.

57. Trotman J, Opat S, Gottlieb D, et al. Zanubrutinib for the treatment of patients with Waldenström macroglobulinemia: 3 years of follow-up. Blood 2020; 136(18):2027–37.

58. An G, Zhou D, Cheng S, et al. A phase II trial of the Bruton tyrosine-kinase inhibitor zanubrutinib (BGB-3111) in patients with relapsed/refractory waldenström macroglobulinemia. Clin Cancer Res 2021;27(20):5492–501.

59. Tam CS, Opat S, D'Sa S, et al. A randomized phase 3 trial of zanubrutinib vs ibrutinib in symptomatic Waldenström macroglobulinemia: the ASPEN study. Blood 2020;136(18):2038–50.

60. Tam CSL, Garcia-Sanz R, Opat S, et al. ASPEN: Long-term follow-up results of a phase 3 randomized trial of zanubrutinib (ZANU) versus ibrutinib (IBR) in patients with Waldenstrom macroglobulinemia (WM). J Clin Oncol 2022;40(16): 7521.

61. Castillo JJ, Kingsley E, Narang M, et al. A phase 2 expanded access study of zanubrutinib (ZANU) in patients (pts) with Waldenström Macroglobulinemia (WM). J Clin Oncol 2022;40(16_suppl):e19522.

62. Owen RG, McCarthy H, Rule S, et al. Acalabrutinib monotherapy in patients with Waldenström macroglobulinemia: a single-arm, multicentre, phase 2 study. Lancet Haematol 2020;7(2):e112–21.

63. Owen R, McCarthy H, Rule S, et al. P1130: acalabrutinib in treatment-naive or relapsed/refractory waldenström macroglobulinemia: 5-year follow-up of a phase 2, single-arm study. HemaSphere 2022;6(S3):1020–1.

64. Sekiguchi N, Rai S, Munakata W, et al. Two-year outcomes of tirabrutinib monotherapy in Waldenstrom's macroglobulinemia. Cancer Sci 2022;113(6):2085–96.

65. Cao X, Jin J, Fu C, et al. Evaluation of orelabrutinib monotherapy in patients with relapsed or refractory Waldenstrom's macroglobulinemia in a single-arm, multicenter, open-label, phase 2 study. Eclinicalmedicine 2022;52:101682.

66. Mato A, Shah N, Jurczak W, et al. Pirtobrutinib in relapsed or refractory B-cell malignancies (BRUIN): a phase 1/2 study. Lancet 2021;397(10277):892–901.

67. Palomba ML, Patel MR, Eyre TA, et al. Efficacy of pirtobrutinib, a highly selective, non-covalent (reversible) BTK inhibitor in relapsed/refractory waldenström macroglobulinemia: results from the phase 1/2 bruin study. Blood 2022; 140(Suppl.1):1.

68. Muhowski EM, Ravikrishnan J, Gordon B, et al. Preclinical evaluation of combination nemtabrutinib and venetoclax in chronic lymphocytic leukemia. J Hematol Oncol 2022;15(1):166.
69. Jiménez C, Chan GG, Xu L, et al. Genomic evolution of ibrutinib-resistant clones in Waldenström macroglobulinaemia. Br J Haematol 2020;189(6):1165–70.
70. Woyach JA, Flinn IW, Awan FT, et al. Efficacy and safety of nemtabrutinib, a wild-type and C481S-mutated Bruton tyrosine kinase inhibitor for B-cell malignancies: updated analysis of the open-label phase 1/2 dose-expansion bellwave-001 study. Blood 2022;140(Supplement 1):7004–6.
71. Gustine JN, Meid K, Dubeau T, et al. Ibrutinib discontinuation in Waldenström macroglobulinemia: etiologies, outcomes, and IgM rebound. Am J Hematol 2018;93(4):511–7.
72. Bond DA, Woyach JA. Targeting BTK in CLL: Beyond Ibrutinib. Curr Hematol Malig Rep 2019;14(3):197–205.
73. Bhat SA, Gambril J, Azali L, et al. Ventricular arrhythmias and sudden death events following acalabrutinib initiation. Blood 2022;140(20):2142–5.
74. Tam CS, Dimopoulos M, Garcia-Sanz R, et al. Pooled safety analysis of zanubrutinib monotherapy in patients with B-cell malignancies. Blood Adv 2022;6(4):1296–308.
75. Kyriakou C. High-dose therapy and hematopoietic stem cell transplantation in waldenström macroglobulinemia. Hematol Oncol Clin North Am 2018;32(5):865–74.
76. Kyriakou C, Canals C, Sibon D, et al. High-dose therapy and autologous stem-cell transplantation in Waldenstrom macroglobulinemia: the Lymphoma Working Party of the European Group for Blood and Marrow Transplantation. J Clin Oncol 2010;28(13):2227–32.
77. Kyriakou C, Canals C, Cornelissen JJ, et al. Allogeneic stem-cell transplantation in patients with Waldenström macroglobulinemia: report from the Lymphoma Working Party of the European Group for Blood and Marrow Transplantation. J Clin Oncol 2010;28(33):4926–34.
78. Chng WJ, Schop RF, Price-Troska T, et al. Gene-expression profiling of Waldenstrom macroglobulinemia reveals a phenotype more similar to chronic lymphocytic leukemia than multiple myeloma. Blood 2006;108(8):2755–63.
79. Castillo JJ, Sarosiek S, Branagan AR, et al. Ibrutinib and venetoclax in previously untreated waldenström macroglobulinemia. Blood 2022;140(Supplement 1):564–5.
80. Vanhaesebroeck B, Perry MWD, Brown JR, et al. PI3K inhibitors are finally coming of age. Nat Rev Drug Discov 2021;20(10):741–69.
81. Tomowiak C, Poulain S, Herbaux C, et al. Obinutuzumab and idelalisib in symptomatic patients with relapsed/refractory Waldenström macroglobulinemia. Blood Adv 2021;5(9):2438–46.
82. Castillo JJ, Gustine JN, Meid K, et al. Idelalisib in Waldenström macroglobulinemia: high incidence of hepatotoxicity. Leuk Lymphoma 2017;58(4):1002–4.
83. Roccaro AM, Sacco A, Jimenez C, et al. C1013G/CXCR4 acts as a driver mutation of tumor progression and modulator of drug resistance in lymphoplasmacytic lymphoma. Blood 2014;123(26):4120–31.
84. Treon SP, Meid K, Hunter ZR, et al. Phase 1 study of ibrutinib and the CXCR4 antagonist ulocuplumab in CXCR4-mutated Waldenström macroglobulinemia. Blood 2021;138(17):1535–9.
85. Treon SP, Buske C, Thomas SK, et al. Preliminary clinical response data from a phase 1b study of mavorixafor in combination with ibrutinib in patients with

waldenström's macroglobulinemia with MYD88 and CXCR4 mutations. Blood 2021;138(Supplement 1):1362.

86. Jalali S, Price-Troska T, Paludo J, et al. Soluble PD-1 ligands regulate T-cell function in Waldenstrom macroglobulinemia. Blood Adv 2018;2(15):1985–97.

87. Ansell SM. PD-1 Is expressed on B-Cells in waldenstrom macroglobulinemia and promotes malignant cell viability and proliferation. Blood 2014;124(21):3015.

88. Kothari J, Eyre TA, Rismani A, et al. Pembrowm: results of a multi-centre phase Ii trial investigating the safety and efficacy of rituximab and pembrolizumab in relapsed/refractory waldenström's macroglobulinaemia. Blood 2022;140(Supplement 1):3624–6.

89. Panayiotidis P, Tumyan G, Thieblemont C, et al. A phase-II study of atezolizumab in combination with obinutuzumab or rituximab for relapsed or refractory mantle cell or marginal zone lymphoma or Waldenström's macroglobulinemia. Leuk Lymphoma 2022;63(5):1–12.

90. Tam C, Cull G, Opat S, et al. An update on safety and preliminary efficacy of highly specific Bruton tyrosine kinase (BTK) Inhibitor zanubrutinib in combination with PD-1 inhibitor tislelizumab in patients with previously treated B-Cell lymphoid malignancies. Blood 2019;134:1594.

91. Othman J, Verner E, Tam C, et al. Severe hemolysis and transfusion reactions after treatment with BGB-3111 and PD-1 antibody for Waldenstrom macroglobulinemia. Haematologica 2018;103(5):E223–5.

92. Amaador K, Vos J, Pals S, et al. Discriminating between Waldenstrom macroglobulinemia and marginal zone lymphoma using logistic LASSO regression. Leuk Lymphoma 2022;63(5):1070–9.

93. Nooka AK, Kaufman JL, Hofmeister CC, et al. Daratumumab in multiple myeloma. Cancer 2019;125(14):2364–82.

94. Castillo JJ, Libby EN, Ansell SM, et al. Multicenter phase 2 study of daratumumab monotherapy in patients with previously treated Waldenström macroglobulinemia. Blood Adv 2020;4(20):5089–92.

95. Puig N, Ocio EM, Jiménez C, et al. Waldenström's Macroglobulinemia Immunophenotype. In: Leblond V, Treon S, Dimopoulos M, editors. Waldenström's macroglobulinemia. Cham: Springer; 2017. https://doi.org/10.1007/978-3-319-22584-5_2.

96. Hamadani M, Radford J, Carlo-Stella C, et al. Final results of a phase 1 study of loncastuximab tesirine in relapsed/refractory B-cell non-Hodgkin lymphoma. Blood 2021;137(19):2634–45.

97. Sterner RC, Sterner RM. CAR-T cell therapy: current limitations and potential strategies. Blood Cancer J 2021;11(4):69.

98. Tbakhi B, Reagan PM. Chimeric antigen receptor (CAR) T-cell treatment for mantle cell lymphoma (MCL). Ther Adv Hematol 2022;13. 20406207221080738.

99. Heyman BM, Tzachanis D, Kipps TJ. Recent advances in CAR T-Cell therapy for patients with chronic lymphocytic leukemia. Cancers 2022;14(7):1715.

100. Palomba ML, Qualls D, Monette S, et al. CD19-directed chimeric antigen receptor T cell therapy in Waldenström macroglobulinemia: a preclinical model and initial clinical experience. J Immunother Cancer 2022;10(2):e004128.

101. Bannerji R, Allan JN, Arnason JE, et al. Clinical activity of REGN1979, a bispecific human, Anti-CD20 x Anti-CD3 antibody, in patients with relapsed/refractory (R/R) B-cell non-hodgkin lymphoma (B-NHL). Blood 2019;134(Supplement_1):762.

102. Longcor J, Callander N, Oliver K, et al. Iopofosine I-131 treatment in late-line patients with relapsed/refractory multiple myeloma post anti-BCMA immunotherapy. Blood Cancer J 2022;12(9):130.

103. Amaador K, Nieuwkerk PT, Minnema MC, et al. Patient preferences regarding treatment options for Waldenström's macroglobulinemia: a discrete choice experiment. Cancer Med 2022;12(3):3376–86.

104. Chen CI, Kouroukis CT, White D, et al. Bortezomib is active in patients with untreated or relapsed Waldenstrom's macroglobulinemia: a phase II study of the National Cancer Institute of Canada Clinical Trials Group. J Clin Oncol 2007; 25(12):1570–5.

105. Dimopoulos M, Tedeschi A, Trotman J, et al. Phase 3 trial of ibrutinib plus rituximab in waldenstrom's macroglobulinemia. N Engl J Med 2018;378(25): 2399–410.

Novel Agents in Waldenström Macroglobulinemia

Shayna Sarosiek, MD[a,b,*], Jorge J. Castillo, MD[a,b]

KEYWORDS

- Waldenström macroglobulinemia • Novel therapies • Targeted therapies
- Immunotherapy

KEY POINTS

- Novel therapies are needed to improve outcomes in patients with Waldenström macroglobulinemia (WM), as WM is incurable with currently available therapies and can severely impact the quality of life of patients with this disease.
- Non-covalent Bruton tyrosine kinase (BTK) inhibitors (eg, pirtobrutinib, nemtabrutinib) seem effective in WM patients who progress on or are intolerant to covalent BTK inhibitors.
- BTK inhibitor-containing regimens (eg, ibrutinib plus venetoclax; acalabrutinib plus bendamustine and rituximab) promise fixed-duration therapy to minimize toxicity and the development of resistance.
- Immunotherapy (eg, antibody-drug conjugates, bispecific antibodies, chimeric antigen receptor T-cell therapy) can potentially achieve deeper and more durable responses in patients with WM.

INTRODUCTION

Waldenström macroglobulinemia (WM) is a rare lymphoplasmacytic lymphoma with specific clinical and pathologic features that distinguish it from other indolent B-cell lymphomas and plasma cell disorders, making the treatment practices unique. Patients with WM typically have a prolonged life expectancy but will require multiple treatments throughout their disease. The current therapeutic landscape for WM includes several treatment options for patients with newly diagnosed WM, such as the Bruton tyrosine kinase (BTK) inhibitors ibrutinib, acalabrutinib, and zanubrutinib, as well as the chemo-immunotherapy regimens bendamustine–rituximab (BR) and cyclophosphamide–rituximab–dexamethasone, and proteasome inhibitor-based regimens. These therapies

a Bing Center for Waldenström Macroglobulinemia, Dana-Farber Cancer Institute, Boston, MA, USA; b Department of Medicine, Harvard Medical School, Boston, MA, USA
* Corresponding author. 450 Brookline Avenue, Mayer 223, Boston, MA 02215.
E-mail address: Shayna_Sarosiek@DFCI.HARVARD.EDU

Hematol Oncol Clin N Am 37 (2023) 751–760
https://doi.org/10.1016/j.hoc.2023.04.001
0889-8588/23/© 2023 Elsevier Inc. All rights reserved.
hemonc.theclinics.com

have high response rates and are generally well tolerated. Still, treatment-emergent adverse effects are present with each therapy, and resistance to these therapies occurs even in the first-line setting. In addition, the response rates and duration of response for these therapies decrease in relapsed and refractory disease. Owing to these limiting factors, additional treatments are being explored with a focus on developing more targeted agents, combination therapies, and in some cases fixed duration therapies to bring patients more effective and less toxic therapies. This review discusses multiple novel agents being developed for treating patients with WM.

BRUTON TYROSINE KINASE INHIBITORS

First- and second-generation covalent BTK inhibitors, such as ibrutinib, acalabrutinib, orelabrutinib, tirabrutinib, and zanubrutinib, have an important role in the treatment of newly diagnosed and relapsed/refractory WM and are part of guideline-directed therapy based on multiple previous publications demonstrating the safety and efficacy of these BTK inhibitors in WM.[1–5] Although they are effective, many patients develop side effects, such as cardiac arrhythmia, bleeding, or rheumatologic symptoms that may require dose reduction or medication changes.[6] In addition, resistance may develop in some patients through multiple potential pathways, such as acquiring phospholipase C $\gamma2$ and BTK mutations (eg, C481).[7,8] In recent years, reversible, noncovalent BTK inhibitors have been developed as a potential treatment option in patients with resistance or intolerance to earlier BTK inhibitors. The initial data have demonstrated efficacy in WM.

Pirtobrutinib

Pirtobrutinib is a novel non-covalent BTK inhibitor recently Food & Drug Administration (FDA)-approved for treating mantle cell lymphoma that inhibits both wild-type and C481-mutant BTK and has proven efficacy in multiple B-cell malignancies, including WM.[9,10] A recent clinical trial enrolled 323 patients with relapsed or refractory B-cell malignancies, including 78 patients with WM with a median number of 3 prior therapies (range 1–11). All patients were treated with single-agent pirtobrutinib across seven dose levels with 200 mg once daily determined to be the recommended phase 2 dosing. Of those patients with WM, 61 (78%) had been previously treated with a BTK inhibitor, and 40 (66%) had progressed on the prior BTK therapy. The major response rate for the 72 evaluable patients was 68% with 17 (24%) very good partial responses (VGPR) and 32 (44%) partial responses (PR). Of those with prior BTK inhibitor exposure, the major response rate was 64%. The median duration of response in the 49 responding patients was not reached at a short median response follow-up of 7.7 months. The most frequent adverse effects in the trial included fatigue, diarrhea, and contusions with the most frequent grade ≥3 adverse event being neutropenia. The discontinuation rate for treatment-related adverse effects was 2%. Owing to these data demonstrating tolerance and efficacy in a heavily pretreated population, additional trials will be pursued, including combination therapies and continued evaluation of the use of pirtobrutinib in patients with prior BTK inhibitor exposure and in patients with treatment naïve disease.

Nemtabrutinib

Nemtabrutinib is another non-covalent BTK inhibitor with efficacy against wild-type and C481-mutated BTK. Early data with this therapy were reported from a clinical trial that enrolled 112 patients, the majority of which had chronic lymphocytic leukemia (CLL) or small lymphocytic lymphoma (SLL) and six patients with WM (NCT03162536).[11]

Individual responses in the patients with WM are not yet available, but of the 57 patients with CLL/SLL, 95% had prior BTK inhibitor exposure, and 63% had a BTK C481 mutation. The overall response rate (ORR) was 56%. The most common drug-related adverse effects were similar to other BTK inhibitors; fatigue, thrombocytopenia, diarrhea, hypertension, and neutropenia, in addition to nausea and the unique effect of dysgeusia in 21% of patients. Grade $\geq$3 adverse effects occurred in 40% of patients, the most common being neutropenia, thrombocytopenia, and lymphocytosis. Additional studies evaluating the continued use of nemtabrutinib (NCT04728893, NCT05347225, and NCT05673460) and another non-covalent BTK inhibitor AS-1763 (NCT05602363) are underway in hopes of developing better tolerated and more effective BTK inhibitors.

BRUTON TYROSINE KINASE DEGRADERS

Additional manners of targeting BTK are also being explored, including BTK degradation, which can potentially overcome intrinsic and acquired BTK resistance in patients with lymphoma. The initial data with DD-03-171, a degrader of BTK inhibitor (BTK), IKFZ1, and IKFZ3, showed the ability to prevent the proliferation of lymphoma cells in vitro and in patient-derived xenografts also demonstrated reduced lymphoma burden and improved overall survival in murine models.[12] Currently, the BTK degraders NX-2127, NX-5948, and BGB-16673 are being explored in patients. NK-2127 degrades BTK and IKZF3 and has immunomodulatory activity with the potential to overcome resistance to currently available covalent and non-covalent BTK inhibitors, as demonstrated in a first-in-human phase 1 trial that has treated 28 patients with relapsed or refractory CLL or B-cell malignancies with NX-2127 at 100 mg daily.[13] All 17 patients with CLL had prior BTKi exposure, and of the 14 CLL samples tested, BTK mutations were found in C481 (29%), L528 (29%), T474 (14%), and V416 (7%). A mean BTK degradation of 86% was seen in all patients, and of the 12 evaluable patients with CLL, the ORR was 33% with evidence that the hematologic response deepens over time (up to 50% at 6 months). Grade $\geq$3 treatment-related adverse effects included neutropenia, anemia, and hypertension. The clinical trial exploring the use of NX-2127 (NCT04830137) continues to recruit and includes patients with CLL and other B-cell malignancies such as WM. NX-5948, a selective degrader of BTK without immunomodulatory activity, has demonstrated in vitro activity and in vivo effects in murine models.[14] Initial studies have also demonstrated central nervous system penetration. Clinical evaluation of this compound is ongoing in patients with relapsed or refractory B-cell malignancies (NCT05131022). Future studies will potentially include patients with central nervous system lymphoma, such as Bing–Neel syndrome. Two phase 1 open-label dose escalation and expansion trials are also ongoing with the BTK degrader BGB-16673 in patients with relapsed or refractory B-cell malignancies (NCT05006716 and NCT05294731). The outcome of this trial will determine the appropriate dose level to use in future phase 2 clinical trials.

BRUTON TYROSINE KINASE INHIBITOR COMBINATIONS

Although BTK inhibitors are effective and generally well-tolerated in WM, the potential for cumulative toxicities and indefinite therapy can be burdensome for patients. Clinical trials are ongoing to evaluate combination and fixed-duration treatment strategies with BTK inhibitors in combination with other therapies.

Based on the data from a phase 2 study of the B-cell leukemia/lymphoma 2 (BCL2) antagonist venetoclax in WM demonstrating an 84% ORR as well as the safety of venetoclax and ibrutinib combination in CLL and mantle cell lymphoma, a clinical trial was designed to evaluate the combination of venetoclax with ibrutinib for a 2-year duration in WM.[15–17] The initial data from this trial show an ORR of 100% with a major response rate of 93% and a median time to minor response of 1.9 months.[18] Eighteen patients (40%) achieved a VGPR and 24 (53%) achieved a PR. The 12-month progression-free survival (PFS) in this trial was 92%. Grade ≥3 adverse events in at least two patients included neutropenia, oral mucositis, tumor lysis, and cardiac arrhythmias. Despite the high hematologic response rates and the previous success of this regimen in other hematologic malignancies, the trial was stopped early due to a high rate of ventricular arrhythmias with four patients (9%) experiencing ventricular arrhythmia and/or cardiac arrest. The exact etiology for the increased risk of arrhythmias in this population compared with patients with other malignancies is unknown. Despite the early cessation of this trial due to toxicity, the trial demonstrated the potential to achieve deep hematologic responses with a finite duration combination of BTK inhibitor and BCL-2 inhibitor, and therefore, additional trials using novel BTK inhibitors, such as pirtobrutinib with venetoclax (NCT05734495), are ongoing.

Another combination therapy with promising early results is the combination of a BTK inhibitor and chemoimmunotherapy, as seen in an ongoing single-arm trial combining six cycles of BR with 12 months of acalabrutinib (NCT04624906).[19] Interim data from this trial reported that eight of the first ten patients had completed all six cycles of BR. All patients had achieved a VGPR at cycle 7. The most common grade ≥3 toxicities were cytopenias with one case each of transaminitis, atrial fibrillation, and infection. Future investigations in this trial will evaluate the rates of minimal residual disease negativity, treatment tolerance, and PFS.

The combination of zanubrutinib, the proteasome inhibitor ixazomib and dexamethasone is being investigated in a phase 2 single-arm study (NCT04463953), and the preliminary results were recently reported.[20] This regimen includes ixazomib and dexamethasone administered for up to six cycles, followed by maintenance therapy every 3 months. Zanubrutinib was administered orally twice daily with all treatment ending after a maximum of 24 months. At the time of data presentation, 20 patients had enrolled in the study and 19 were evaluable for response. Eight patients had achieved a VGPR (42%), ten had a PR (53%), and one had a minor response (5%) for an ORR of 100% and a major response rate of 95%. The median time to minor response was 1.1 months. Two patients achieved minimal residual disease negativity. Grade ≥3 serious adverse events of rash and neutropenia were observed in two patients. Additional results from this trial will be reported in the future. Another proteasome inhibitor-based clinical trial is ongoing to explore the use of carfilzomib in combination with ibrutinib compared with ibrutinib alone in WM (NCT04263480). These combination trials offer the potential for a fixed-duration therapy with deep hematologic responses.

C-X-C CHEMOKINE RECEPTOR TYPE 4 TARGETING AGENTS

C-X-C chemokine receptor type 4 (CXCR4) mutations are present in approximately 40% of patients with WM and may serve as another potential therapeutic target.[21] This additional mutation is associated with a longer time to hematologic response, decreased rates of major responses, and shorter PFS in patients treated with BTK inhibitors.[4,22] One CXCR4 antagonist, ulocuplumab, was initially explored in combination with ibrutinib.[23] Ulocuplumab was administered every other week during cycles 2 to 6. Ibrutinib was given daily with the intention of continuing ibrutinib indefinitely in the setting of continued disease response and tolerance of therapy. In this study, 12 patients were evaluable for response with 100% overall and major response rate. The time to minor and major responses were 0.9 and 1.2 months, respectively. Compared with historical data, the time to response, depth of response, and PFS compared favorably to single-agent ibrutinib in patients without CXCR4 mutations. Following this trial, an additional trial investigating the use of the CXCR4 antagonist mavorixafor was initiated.[24] Mavorixafor 200 to 600 mg orally once daily was given with ibrutinib, and preliminary data after 10 patients were enrolled showed an ORR of 100%, with four of eight patients achieving a major response. This clinical trial is now closed to enrollment, and outcome data are expected in the near future. Despite the efficacy and safety of these agents in combination with ibrutinib, the additional development of these agents is not currently being pursued, but CXCR4 antagonists may still play a role in the future therapy for WM.

OTHER TARGETED AGENTS

Continued exploration of the B-cell receptor and nuclear factor kappa B (NF-κB) pathways has led to the development of additional targeted therapies. Mucosa-associated lymphoid tissue translocation protein 1 (MALT1), when dysregulated, is known to contribute to the development of lymphoid malignancies and has emerged as a potential target in lymphomas such as WM which rely on NF-κB pathway upregulation.[25]

JNJ-67856633, a potent, selective MALT-1 inhibitor showing preclinical activity in activated B-cell diffuse large B-cell lymphoma, is being explored in combination with ibrutinib (NCT04876092) and in combination with a novel BTK inhibitor JNJ-6426481 (NCT04657224) in patients with non-Hodgkin lymphomas.[26] SGR-1505 and ONO-7018, additional MALT1 inhibitors, are also actively being studied in phase 1 open-label clinical trials evaluating these drugs' safety and pharmacologic characteristics in patients with relapsed or refractory B-cell malignancies (NCT05544019 and NCT05515406).

Another small molecule inhibitor currently in development is emavusertib (CA-4948), an inhibitor of interleukin-1 receptor-associated kinase 4 (IRAK4). IRAK4 is part of the myddosome signaling pathway known to be dysregulated in WM. Hence, an ongoing phase 1 clinical trial (NCT03328078) enrolling patients with relapsed or refractory hematologic malignancies, including WM. Preliminary data have reported three patients with WM enrolled in the trial with two of the three patients achieving a PR.[27] Recruitment for this trial is ongoing. Future studies may also be pursued in Bing–Neel syndrome, as early data have shown that emavusertib crosses the blood-brain barrier, and some central nervous system tumors, such as primary central nervous system lymphoma, have demonstrated susceptibility to this compound in laboratory testing.[28]

IMMUNOTHERAPIES
Chimeric Antigen Receptor T Cells

Several new therapies in the immunotherapy field have been approved for multiple myeloma and lymphoma. One of these therapies, chimeric antigen receptor (CAR) T-cell therapy, is actively being investigated in WM. The initial preclinical data with a CAR T-cell therapy targeted against the CD19 antigen demonstrated activity in WM cells in vitro and in vivo murine models of WM.[29] These data were followed by a report of three patients with relapsed and refractory WM treated with CD19-directed CAR T-cell therapy in clinical trials (NCT03085173 and NCT00466531). All three patients responded to CAR T-cell treatment with one attaining a minimal residual disease-negative complete response. However, these responses had limited durability as all patients relapsed between 3 and 26 months. Additional data from these two clinical trials are not yet available, but the studies are ongoing.

A large clinical trial using brexucabtagene autoleucel, a cluster of differentiation 19 (CD19) CAR T-cell construct, has FDA approval for treating relapsed or refractory mantle cell lymphoma, and B-cell precursor adult lymphocytic leukemia is currently recruiting patients with WM. It will provide additional data on the safety of this construct in WM (NCT05537766). In the initial trials that led to the approval of brexucabtagene autoleucel, the most common non-hematologic grade ≥3 adverse effects included fever/febrile neutropenia, hypotension, infection, hypoxia, cytokine release syndrome, and neurologic toxicity with the latter two adverse effects being frequently associated with CAR T-cell therapy.[30,31] Most patients also developed leukopenia, neutropenia, lymphopenia, thrombocytopenia, and anemia.

An additional CAR T-cell product with preliminary data in non-Hodgkin lymphoma is MB-106, a cluster of differentiation 20 (CD20)-targeted CAR T with M-1BB, and CD28 costimulatory domains. An ORR of 94% was reported in the initial 16 patients with relapsed or refractory B-cell non-Hodgkin lymphoma treated with this construct. Less than half of patients (n = 7, 44%) developed cytokine release syndrome with all cases being grade 1 or 2 and immune effector cell-associated neurotoxicity syndrome in only one patient (6%), which compares favorably to other CAR T-cell constructs. A large clinical trial with MB-106 is ongoing (NCT05360238) and will include patients with WM. Data from the first two patients with WM treated with this construct were previously presented and showed a hematologic response in both patients.[32]

Antibody-Drug Conjugates

Another novel immunotherapy being investigated in WM is loncastuximab tesirine, a CD19-directed antibody-drug conjugate. Loncastuximab tesirine has been FDA-approved for use in patients with relapsed or refractory diffuse large B-cell lymphoma based on phase 1 data demonstrating an ORR of 43%, 47%, and 79% in diffuse large B-cell lymphoma, mantle cell lymphoma, and follicular lymphoma, respectively.[33] Additional phase 2 data in diffuse large B-cell lymphoma reported a response rate of 48% and a complete response rate of 24% with the most common grade ≥3 treatment-related adverse events in these trials being neutropenia, thrombocytopenia, and elevation in gamma-glutamyltransferase. Based on response rates and tolerance of this therapy in both aggressive and indolent B-cell lymphomas with CD19 expression, it was thought that the CD19 expression seen on lymphocytes and plasma cells in WM might make this disease susceptible to treatment with loncastuximab tesirine.[34,35] An ongoing clinical trial (NCT05190705) should provide information on the efficacy and safety of this drug in WM.

Bispecific Antibodies

In recent years, bispecific antibodies, particularly those with the B-cell specific surface antigen CD20 and the T-cell surface antigen CD3 binding sites, have been successfully explored in non-Hodgkin lymphoma. Mosunetuzumab, a CD20 and CD3 bispecific antibody, was recently granted FDA approval for treating advanced follicular lymphoma. Ongoing trials are exploring the use of this bispecific as well as glofitamab, epcoritamab, and odronextamab in non-Hodgkin lymphoma.[36] To date, data are not available for the use of these products in WM. However, additional evaluation of these therapies in WM is warranted and the development of these clinical trials is underway.

Phospholipid-Drug Conjugates

Iopofosine I-131 (previously known as CLR131) is a small-molecule phospholipid-drug conjugate. This radiopharmaceutical is designed to deliver a radioisotope, iodine-131, directly to cancer cells. This drug has been granted Fast Track Designation and

Table 1
Selected prospective clinical trials evaluating novel agents in Waldenström macroglobulinemia

ClinicalTrials.Gov ID	Agents	Phase	Setting
NCT02952508	Iopofosine 131	II	RR
NCT03620903	Ibrutinib, bortezomib, rituximab	II	TN
NCT04061512	Ibrutinib, rituximab vs DRC	III	TN
NCT04263480	Ibrutinib, carfilzomib vs ibrutinib	III	TN
NCT04463953	Zanubrutinib, ixazomib, dexamethasone	II	TN
NCT04624906	Acalabrutinib, bendamustine, rituximab	II	TN
NCT04728893	Nemtabrutinib	II	RR
NCT05099471	Venetoclax, rituximab vs. DRC	II	TN
NCT05190705	Loncastuximab tesirine	II	RR
NCT05360238	MB-106	II	RR
NCT05537766	Brexucabtagene autoleucel	II	RR
NCT05734495	Pirtobrutinib, venetoclax	II	RR

Abbreviations: DRC, dexamethasone, rituximab, cyclophosphamide; RR, relapsed or refractory; TN, treatment-naïve.

Orphan Drug Designation by the US Food and Drug Administration based on data from the CLOVER-1 phase 2 trial. This initial trial enrolled patients with multiple indolent lymphomas, including six patients with WM.[37] The ORR in these patients was 100% with 83% major responses, including one complete response. The median time to initial response was 48 days. The median duration of response has yet to be reached. The primary treatment-emergent adverse events were cytopenias and fatigue. A trial dedicated to WM is now ongoing (NCT02952508).

Table 1 lists selected clinical trials with novel agents in patients with WM.

SUMMARY

There are several safe and effective options to treat patients with WM. However, WM remains incurable using standard therapies; therefore, agents with novel and non-cross-resistant mechanisms of action are needed. A wide variety of targeted agents and immunotherapies are undergoing clinical development in patients with WM aimed at improving the response and survival of these patients while minimizing adverse events. These newer agents are likely to chisel the treatment landscape of WM. Multi-institutional efforts and energetic patient participation are needed to complete these clinical trials.

CLINICS CARE POINTS

- Multiple effective therapies for WM exist, but novel therapies are needed due to the long life expectancy of patients with WM, as well as the risk of disease relapse and development of treatment resistance.

CONTRIBUTIONS

S. Sarosiek and J.J. Castillo: Conception, writing, and final approval of the article.

DISCLOSURES

J.J. Castillo received research funds and/or honoraria from Abbvie, United States, AstraZeneca, BeiGene, China, Cellectar, Janssen, United States, Kite, LOXO, Pharmacyclics, United States, Roche, Switzerland, and TG Therapeutics, United States. S. Sarosiek received research funds and/or honoraria from Beigene, Cellectar, and ADC Therapeutics.

REFERENCES

1. Owen RG, McCarthy H, Rule S, et al. Acalabrutinib monotherapy in patients with Waldenstrom macroglobulinemia: a single-arm, multicentre, phase 2 study. Lancet Haematol 2020;7(2):e112–21.
2. Sekiguchi N, Rai S, Munakata W, et al. A multicenter, open-label, phase II study of tirabrutinib (ONO/GS-4059) in patients with Waldenstrom's macroglobulinemia. Cancer Sci 2020;111(9):3327–37.
3. Tam CS, Opat S, D'Sa S, et al. A randomized phase 3 trial of zanubrutinib versus ibrutinib in symptomatic waldenstrom macroglobulinemia:the aspen study. Blood 2020;136(18):2038–50.
4. Treon SP, Gustine J, Meid K, et al. Ibrutinib monotherapy in symptomatic, treatment-naive patients with waldenstrom macroglobulinemia. J Clin Oncol 2018;36(27):2755–61.
5. Treon SP, Tripsas CK, Meid K, et al. Ibrutinib in previously treated Waldenstrom's macroglobulinemia. N Engl J Med 2015;372(15):1430–40.
6. Sarosiek S, Gustine JN, Flynn CA, et al. Dose reductions in patients with Waldenstrom macroglobulinaemia treated with ibrutinib. Br J Haematol 2023. https://doi.org/10.1111/bjh.18643.
7. Xu L, Tsakmaklis N, Yang G, et al. Acquired mutations associated with ibrutinib resistance in Waldenstrom macroglobulinemia. Blood 2017;129(18):2519–25.
8. Stephens DM, Byrd JC. Resistance to Bruton tyrosine kinase inhibitors: the Achilles heel of their success story in lymphoid malignancies. Blood 2021;138(13):1099–109.
9. Palomba ML, Patel MR, Eyre TA, et al. Efficacy of pirtobrutinib, a highly selective, non-covalent (Reversible) BTK Inhibitor in relapsed/refractory waldenström macroglobulinemia: results from the phase 1/2 BRUIN study. Blood 2022;140(Supplement 1):557–60.
10. Mato AR, Shah NN, Jurczak W, et al. Pirtobrutinib in relapsed or refractory B-cell malignancies (BRUIN): a phase 1/2 study. Lancet 2021;397(10277):892–901.
11. Woyach J.A., Flinn I.W., Awan F.T., et al., Efficacy and safety of nemtabrutinib, a wild-type and C481S-mutated bruton tyrosine kinase inhibitor for B-Cell malignancies: updated analysis of the open-label phase 1/2 dose-expansion bellwave-001 study, *Blood*, 140 (Supplement 1), 2022, 7004–7006.
12. Dobrovolsky D, Wang ES, Morrow S, et al. Bruton tyrosine kinase degradation as a therapeutic strategy for cancer. Blood 2019;133(9):952–61.
13. Mato AR, Wierda WG, Ai WZ, et al. NX-2127-001, a First-in-Human Trial of NX-2127, a Bruton's tyrosine kinase-targeted protein degrader, in patients with relapsed or refractory chronic lymphocytic leukemia and B-Cell malignancies. Blood 2022;140(1):2329–32.
14. Robbins DW, Noviski M, Rountree R, et al. Nx-5948, a selective degrader of BTK with activity in preclinical models of hematologic and brain malignancies. Blood 2021;138(1):2251.

15. Castillo JJ, Allan JN, Siddiqi T, et al. Venetoclax in previously treated waldenstrom macroglobulinemia. J Clin Oncol 2022;40(1):63–71.

16. Jain N, Keating M, Thompson P, et al. Ibrutinib and venetoclax for first-line treatment of CLL. N Engl J Med 2019;380(22):2095–103.

17. Tam CS, Anderson MA, Pott C, et al. Ibrutinib plus Venetoclax for the Treatment of Mantle-Cell Lymphoma. N Engl J Med 2018;378(13):1211–23.

18. Castillo JJ, Sarosiek S, Branagan AR, et al. Ibrutinib and venetoclax in previously untreated Waldenström macroglobulinemia. Blood 2022;140(1):564–5.

19. Berinstein NL, Klein G, Welsh K, et al. Next generation BTK inhibitor acalabrutinib with bendamustine-rituximab in first line waldenstrom's macroglobulinemia: the brawm study. Blood 2022;(1):9383–4.

20. Yu Y, Yi S, Wenjie X, et al. Zanubrutinib plus ixazomib and dexamethasone for newly diagnosed symptomatic waldenström macroglobulinemia: a prospective, phase II study. Blood 2022;140(1):3587–8.

21. Hunter ZR, Xu L, Yang G, et al. The genomic landscape of Waldenstrom macroglobulinemia is characterized by highly recurring MYD88 and WHIM-like CXCR4 mutations, and small somatic deletions associated with B-cell lymphomagenesis. Blood 2014;123(11):1637–46.

22. Treon SP, Meid K, Gustine J, et al. Long-term follow-up of ibrutinib monotherapy in symptomatic, previously treated patients with waldenstrom macroglobulinemia. J Clin Oncol 2021;39(6):565–75.

23. Treon SP, Meid K, Hunter ZR, et al. Phase 1 study of ibrutinib and the CXCR4 antagonist ulocuplumab in CXCR4-mutated Waldenstrom macroglobulinemia. Blood 2021;138(17):1535–9.

24. Treon S.P., Buske C., Thomas S.K., et al., Preliminary clinical response data from a phase 1b study of mavorixafor in combination with ibrutinib in patients with waldenström's macroglobulinemia with MYD88 and CXCR4 mutations. Blood, 138 (Supplement 1), 2021, 1362.

25. Yin W, Zhe N, Placzek A, et al. Identification of potent paracaspase MALT1 inhibitors for hematological malignancies. Blood 2020;136(Supplement 1):30.

26. Philippar U, Attar RM, Lu T, et al. Discovery of JNJ-67856633: a novel, first-in-class MALT1 protease inhibitor for the treatment of b cell lymphomas. Cancer Res 2020;80(Supplement 16):5690.

27. Nowakowski GS, Leslie LA, Younes A, et al. Safety, pharmacokinetics and activity of CA-4948, an IRAK4 inhibitor, for treatment of patients with relapsed or refractory hematologic malignancies: results from the phase 1 study. Blood 2020; 136(Supplement 1):44–5.

28. Von Roemeling C, Doonan BP, Klippel K, et al. Oral IRAK-4 inhibitor CA-4948 is blood-brain barrier penetrant and has single-agent activity against CNS lymphoma and melanoma brain metastases. Clin Cancer Res 2023. https://doi.org/10.1158/1078-0432.CCR-22-1682.

29. Palomba ML, Qualls D, Monette S, et al. CD19-directed chimeric antigen receptor T cell therapy in Waldenstrom macroglobulinemia: a preclinical model and initial clinical experience. J Immunother Cancer 2022;10(2). https://doi.org/10.1136/jitc-2021-004128.

30. Shah BD, Ghobadi A, Oluwole OO, et al. KTE-X19 for relapsed or refractory adult B-cell acute lymphoblastic leukaemia: phase 2 results of the single-arm, open-label, multicentre ZUMA-3 study. Lancet 2021;398(10299):491–502.

31. Wang M, Munoz J, Goy A, et al. KTE-X19 CAR T-cell therapy in relapsed or refractory mantle-cell lymphoma. N Engl J Med 2020;382(14):1331–42.

32. Mustang Bio Announces Phase 1/2 Clinical Trial Data of MB-106, a First-in-Class CD20-targeted, Autologous CAR T Cell Therapy, to be Presented at 11th International Workshop for Waldenstrom's Macroglobulinemia. Available at: https://ir.mustangbio.com/news-events/press-releases/detail/150/mustang-bio-announces-phase-12-clinical-trial-data-of. Accessed March 22, 2023.

33. Hamadani M, Radford J, Carlo-Stella C, et al. Final results of a phase 1 study of loncastuximab tesirine in relapsed/refractory B-cell non-hodgkin lymphoma. Blood 2020. https://doi.org/10.1182/blood.2020007512.

34. Morice WG, Chen D, Kurtin PJ, et al. Novel immunophenotypic features of marrow lymphoplasmacytic lymphoma and correlation with Waldenstrom's macroglobulinemia. Mod Pathol 2009;22(6):807–16.

35. Rosado FG, Morice WG, He R, et al. Immunophenotypic features by multiparameter flow cytometry can help distinguish low grade B-cell lymphomas with plasmacytic differentiation from plasma cell proliferative disorders with an unrelated clonal B-cell process. Br J Haematol 2015;169(3):368–76.

36. Falchi L, Vardhana SA, Salles GA. Bispecific antibodies for the treatment of B-cell lymphoma: promises, unknowns, and opportunities. Blood 2023;141(5):467–80.

37. Ailawadhi S, Chanan-Khan A, Peterson JL, et al. Treatment free remission (TFR) and overall response rate (ORR) results in patients with relapsed/refractory Waldenstrom's macroglobulinemia (WM) treated with CLR 131. J Clin Oncol 2021;39(15):7561.

Investigation and Management of Immunoglobulin M– and Waldenström-Associated Peripheral Neuropathies

Oliver Tomkins, BMBS, MRCP[a], Veronique Leblond, MD, PhD[b],
Michael P. Lunn, FRCP, PhD[c], Karine Viala, MD[d],
Damien Roos-Weil, MD, PhD[b], Shirley D'Sa, FRCP, FRCPath, MD(Res)[a],*

KEYWORDS

- IgM neuropathy • Paraproteinemic neuropathy • Anti-MAG • CANOMAD

KEY POINTS

- Immunoglobulin M (IgM)-associated peripheral neuropathies are a heterogeneous group of disorders, which together represent most of the cases of paraproteinemic neuropathy.
- Anti-myelin-associated glycoprotein neuropathy constitutes half of the IgM-related cases, and antibody-negative IgM demyelinating neuropathy, multifocal motor neuropathy with conduction block, light chain amyloid neuropathy, cryoglobulinemic neuropathy, and CANOMAD syndrome form most of the remainder.
- Patients with a progressive disability could be treated with rituximab-based therapy, with or without additional chemotherapy.

INTRODUCTION

The immunoglobulin M (IgM)-associated peripheral neuropathies (PNs) are a heterogeneous group of disorders that can result in significant disability, and together they represent most of the cases of paraproteinemic neuropathy.[1] IgM-PNs are associated with a monoclonal gammopathy of undetermined significance (MGUS)—in this

[a] Department of Haematology, Centre for Waldenströms Macroglobulinaemia and Related Conditions, University College London Hospitals NHS Foundation Trust, 250 Euston Road, London NW1 2PG, UK; [b] Department of Haematology, Sorbonne University and Pitié Salpêtrière Hospital, 47-83 Bd de l'Hôpital, Paris 75013, France; [c] National Hospital for Neurology and Neurosurgery, Queen Square, London WC1N 3BG, UK; [d] Department of Clinical Neurophysiology, Sorbonne University and Pitié Salpêtrière Hospital, 47-83 Bd de l'Hôpital, Paris 75013, France
* Corresponding author.
E-mail address: s.dsa@nhs.net
Twitter: @tomkinsoliver (O.T.)

Hematol Oncol Clin N Am 37 (2023) 761–776
https://doi.org/10.1016/j.hoc.2023.04.007
0889-8588/23/© 2023 Elsevier Inc. All rights reserved.
hemonc.theclinics.com

context, perhaps better termed monoclonal gammopathy of neurological significance—or Waldenström macroglobulinemia (WM).[2,3] More rarely, IgM-PN occurs with other chronic B-cell disorders secreting IgM.

The pathophysiologic mechanisms through which the underlying clonal disorder causes neuropathy are manifold and include (1) autoantibody activity of the IgM directed to different antigenic components of the peripheral nerves, (2) the physicochemical properties of the circulating IgM resulting in cryoglobulinemic vasculitis, (3) the deposition of amyloid causing direct neural insult, and (4) neoplastic infiltration of peripheral nerves, known as neurolymphomatosis. The various mechanisms determine different clinically distinct presentations. Appropriate investigations may help clinicians identify the neuropathy mechanism to adapt the therapeutic strategy to the patient.

Given the significant background rates of both neuropathies and paraproteinemia, their coexistence in an individual patient does not immediately infer causality. However, an IgM paraprotein is of unique immunogenicity and is often significant. At the heart of the diagnostic approach lies the collaborative work and experience of the hematologist and neurologist in the clinic.

INCIDENCE AND PREVALENCE

IgM paraproteins and neuropathies are common in an older population where the median age of onset of paraproteinemic neuropathy is 59 years.[4] The population prevalence of monoclonal gammopathy is estimated to be 3.2% in persons older than 50 years, increasing steadily with age. IgG paraproteins account for the majority; IgM paraprotein comprises 16.9% of the overall total.[5] MGUS exceeds WM as the underlying diagnosis by at least 3:1,[6] probably because MGUS is more common. The prevalence of disease-related IgM-PN in patients with WM is 13% to 22%.[7,8] For IgM MGUS, estimates of an associated IgM-PN are 15% to 31%, but the latter is likely to be an overestimate.[9] A recent analysis with a 20% prevalence of PN in patients with IgM monoclonal gammopathies identified that a quarter of the "IgM-PN" cases had other causes, resulting in an IgM-PN prevalence of 15%.[6] Thus, neuropathies associated with IgM paraproteins are frequently encountered, but a causal link is not always present, and other causes of neuropathy or disability should be sought.

PROGNOSIS

Most patients remain functionally able and independent even after many years, and most will not come to require treatment.[10] However, some will progress, and the varying neuropathologies have differing clinical consequences (eg, progressive autonomic failure alongside sensory and motor deficits in light chain (AL) amyloid result in specific disabilities). Some will need mobility aids, analgesia, and cardiovascular support.

SPECIFIC IMMUNOGLOBULIN M AUTOANTIBODY REACTIVITY
Immunoglobulin M Anti-myelin-Associated Glycoprotein Paraproteinemic Peripheral Neuropathy

The clinical phenotype of anti-MAG neuropathy is classic and easily recognisable. Patients are typically men and in their seventh decade (median 62.6 years).[11] Patients present with progressive, symmetric distal sensory loss in the feet associated with early unsteadiness and frequently a complex tremor. The tremor is postural and has both cerebellar and peripheral features, with a side-to-side finger tremor and some jerkiness, potentially disabling.[12] Anti-MAG PN is usually painless, and positive sensory symptoms include "tightness" or "aching." As a result of the sensory loss, patients walk with a broad-based gait with foot misplacement and experience unsteadiness predominantly in the dark. Motor weakness is a late feature and predominantly involves the distal legs.

On examination, sensory neuropathy with reduced or absent reflexes is found. Defining features are a tremor of the upper limbs, little or no wasting of muscles, and a typical sensory loss. Pinprick is reduced distally in the lower limbs, joint position sense is minimally impaired, but vibration sensation is often reduced to the hips or even the costal margin.[13]

Typical nerve conduction study (NCS) findings demonstrate a patchy demyelinating neuropathy, with very prolonged distal motor latencies compared with the slowing of the main motor trunk, resulting in a terminal latency index of less than 0.25 in some but not necessarily all tested nerves.[11,14]

Anti-MAG activity is part of the innate antibody repertoire. Disease-relevant IgM anti-MAG activity can be detected in the serum using one of several techniques, usually enzyme-linked immunosorbent assay–based. Anti-MAG antibodies cross-react with sulfoglucuronyl paragloboside and sulfoglucuronosyl lactosaminyl paragloboside, gangliosides that all display the common carbohydrate HNK-1 epitope.[1,15,16] Although there are various ways that these antibodies are reported, anti-MAG activity is much more likely to be relevant when the levels of activity are reported as "strongly positive" (Buhlmann titer units > 70,000).[17–19] Finding an anti-MAG antibody does not mandate a diagnosis of an anti-MAG neuropathy; the clinical and electrophysiologic picture must also be consistent, with the antibody result considered confirmatory. A nerve biopsy is usually not performed, as the clinical and electrophysiologic features associated with an anti-MAG antibody are usually diagnostic. When performed, widely spaced myelin (widening of the intraperiod line on electron microscopy) is pathognomic.[15,20]

The natural history is most usually indolent and slowly progressive, with favourable long-term outcomes even without treatment in some. Disability rates at 5 years from diagnosis have been quoted at 16%, increasing to 22% to -24% at 10 years and 50% at 15 years.[4,10] Half of patients do not require treatment. The mere presence of anti-MAG neuropathy is not an indication for treatment, whereas measurably progressive patient disability is.[2] More data regarding the treatment of anti-MAG neuropathy are needed. Therapy is best considered stabilizing, as clinical improvement is less common and typically limited.[2] A Cochrane meta-analysis concluded that there is an insufficient evidence base to support specific treatments[21] and that intravenous immunoglobulin (IVIg) had a statistically, but probably not clinically, significant short-term effect with rapidly waning efficacy. Meta-analysis of 2 rituximab studies demonstrated a benefit not found in the underpowered individual studies. The placebo-controlled RiMAG[22] study (375 mg/m^2 weekly for 4 weeks) found no significant difference in sensory scores but significant improvement in disability scales at 12 months. Self-assessment by patients found that 26% experienced improvement and 52% stabilization following rituximab. With placebo, figures were 3% and 36%, respectively. A second study found a significant improvement in the time to walk 10 meters in patients randomized to rituximab over placebo.[23]

Transient worsening with rituximab has been reported, attributed to IgM flares in the setting of WM.[24] Despite the paucity of evidence, rituximab is recommended for progressive anti-MAG neuropathy, especially when associated with MGUS.[2] A short disease duration (<2 years and probably <5 years) and active progression at treatment time favourably predict response to therapy.[7]

In severe and rapid progressive anti-MAG neuropathy, adding chemotherapy to rituximab can be an option leading to a shorter response time. In a retrospective study in

64 patients, improvement at 1 year of the modified Rankin score rates were 46% and 18% in the immunochemotherapy group and rituximab group of patients, respectively, with a median time to response of 8 and 13 months (p = 0.023).[25] The Bruton tyrosine kinase (BTK) inhibitor ibrutinib also has some early promising reports, with several patients exhibiting PN stabilization or improvement; this includes subjective reports in 13 patients and objective reports in 3 patients with the MYD88[L265P] mutation, most previously treated with rituximab.[26–28]

Neuropathies with Immunoglobulin M Activity Directed to Other Peripheral Nerve Epitopes

Gangliosides are present on the surface of many cells but are elaborated on nervous system cells with more than 100 classes detected. They present a somewhat carbohydrate antigenic target, as the glycoprotein MAG mentioned earlier, and likewise can be targeted by IgM antibodies.

Multifocal Motor Neuropathy with Conduction Block

IgM paraprotein with autoantibody activity against ganglioside GM1 is associated with a progressive motor phenotype with distal, asymmetric upper limb weakness, a characteristic distinct from other IgM-PN. Sometimes there is combined anti-GD1b activity with high laboratory titers implicating the paraprotein component. Neurophysiology demonstrates a demyelinating neuropathy characterized by multiple conduction blocks and normal sensory action potentials. In multifocal motor neuropathy with conduction block (MMNCB), individual nerves can be identified with a mononeuritis multiplex presentation.[29]

Anti-GM1 IgM is seen in 40% of all cases of MMNCB. GM1 serves an important function in maintaining motor nerve function. Although anti-GM1 antibodies are identifiable in healthy individuals, in the presence of a suspected immune motor neuropathy, a high-titer anti-GM1 IgM is 85% specific.[30] IVIg has an established role in managing nonparaproteinemic MMNCB, and multiple randomized controlled trials have demonstrated a clear benefit.[31] A Cochrane meta-analysis concluded a 76% improvement in muscle strength with IVIg versus 4% in placebo.[32] Most patients depend on maintenance IVIg to maintain muscle strength. Although there is an improvement with evidence of remyelination and reinnervation, there is still progressive axonal loss over time.[33] If IVIg is ineffective, suppression of the IgM clone is worthwhile, although unsupported by evidence.

CANOMAD Syndrome

This is an acronym for the very rare condition of chronic ataxic neuropathy, ophthalmoplegia, IgM paraprotein, cold agglutinins, and disialosyl antibodies. Patients are typically in their seventh decade of life (median age 62 years) and 80% are men.[34] IgM targets disialosyl epitopes on gangliosides, GD1b/GD3/GT1b/GC1b.[34,35] Half of the cases have antidisialosyl IgM that reacts to all 4 epitopes.[34] These gangliosides predominate in the dorsal root ganglia and oculomotor nerves, resulting in a clinical presentation with chronic ataxic neuropathy and ophthalmoplegia. The acronym can be restrictive, as not all features are always present; ophthalmoplegia is present in only half of the cases and cold agglutinins in a third.[34] CANDA, chronic ataxic neuropathy with disialosyl antibodies, has been suggested as an alternative.[36] A recent study identified that the main clinical features were sensory symptoms with ataxia and paraesthesia (100%), motor weakness (42%), ophthalmoplegia (42%), and bulbar symptoms (12%). Cold agglutinins were identified in 13 (30%) patients. Electrophysiologic studies showed a predominant demyelinating pattern with low or absent sensory action potentials and slow motor conduction velocities. An axonal pattern is rare.[34] Excluding infiltrative causes in patients with ophthalmoplegia and other cranial nerve palsies is imperative.

CANOMAD syndrome is responsive to IVIg in 40% to 60%[34,37] and therapeutic plasmapheresis in 50% of cases,[34] in retrospective analyses. Improvement with rituximab-based therapy has an efficacy of 53%, used in patients refractory to IVIg. It can be readministered efficaciously in patients who progress after a period of improvement or stability, although no randomized evidence exists.[34]

Physicochemical properties of the immunoglobulin M

Cryoglobulinemic vasculitis. Monoclonal IgM can be associated with type I and type II cryoglobulinemia. IgM monoclonal type I cryoglobulin deposits result in vascular occlusion, whereas type II results in small and medium vasculitis. There is a greater proportion of peripheral neuropathy in type II.[38,39] Patients with cryoglobulinemic vasculitis present with painful distal sensory neuropathy with burning, shooting pains, and deep aching; however, it can present with asymmetrical presentations or multifocal mononeuropathy. Systemic clues are livedo reticularis and lower limb ulceration, with multiple small and "punched out" ulcers. Renal involvement and polyarthralgia are rarer. PN is the most frequent symptom after skin purpura.[38,40–42]

Neurophysiology demonstrates an axonal length-dependent sensorimotor neuropathy, often with an asymmetrical component. A nerve biopsy is required in cases of isolated cryoglobulinemia without cutaneous or renal features. The most affected sensory nerve, typically the sural or superficial peroneal, can be identified neurophysiologically. Typical findings are of large fiber degeneration without evidence of regeneration, and alongside are common features of vasculitis with inflammatory infiltrates around the vessels. Intravascular cryoglobulin deposition in vasa nervorum is described.[43]

Mild symptoms may abate with cold prevention, but in cases of rapidly progressive neuropathies plasma exchange may temporize critical symptoms. Definitive treatment should be directed at the underlying clone. High-dose corticosteroids and rituximab are first-line treatments. After rituximab failure, alkylating agents in combination with rituximab and other treatments can be used.[44]

Light chain amyloid neuropathy. IgM-associated AL amyloidosis accounts for 5% to 7% of all amyloidosis. In IgM-related AL amyloidosis, direct axonal nerve damage occurs through amyloid fibril deposition in endoneurium and endoneurial vessels, resulting in neuropathy. It represents 6% of cases of IgM-PN.[6,8] Neuropathy is the presenting feature in 15% of all AL amyloid cases and 28% of IgM-related AL amyloid.[45,46] Compared with non-IgM amyloidosis, the proportion of lambda light chain is small with a relatively low free light chain level. Patients have rapidly progressive length-dependent painful PN with paraesthesia, burning, and allodynia. Asymmetric distribution is seen in 50%.[47] Cranial nerve involvement and a mononeuritis multiplex have been described.[48] The neurophysiology shows progressive axonal neuropathy. Initially, there is a small fiber neuropathy resulting in autonomic dysfunction,[49,50] but with time there is large fiber involvement. Small fiber neuropathies are distal, symmetrical, purely sensory, and painful. The pain is characteristically burning and very prominent at night, often disturbing sleep. No signs are found on examination, as the tendon reflexes and joint position, vibration, and sometimes pinprick sensation are preserved. Standard neurophysiology testing is also normal, but thermal thresholding (quantitative sensory testing) or Sudoscan can demonstrate abnormalities.[51] Other findings consistent with AL amyloidosis should be sought, for example, orthostatic hypotension, erectile dysfunction, diarrhoea, proteinuria, and cardiac involvement.[6,47]

Incidental MGUS can occur with non-AL amyloidosis causes, most commonly hereditary transthyretin amyloidosis.[47] The diagnosis of amyloidosis is histological. Attempts should initially focus on least invasive biopsies, such as abdominal fat aspiration, a rectal biopsy, and/or trephine biopsy, with Congo red staining. A nerve biopsy may be necessary when the index of suspicion remains high.[2,47] Where biopsy is inconclusive or not feasible, a radiolabelled serum amyloid-P scan with a 90% sensitivity is used when available. Although unable to demonstrate nervous deposition, it can confirm the presence of visceral amyloid deposits to be biopsied.[52] Any biopsy confirming the presence of amyloid deposition should be sent for typing to determine the precursor protein and accurately diagnose the amyloidosis subtype before initiating treatment.

Therapy for IgM-related AL amyloidosis is urgently directed at the underlying clone to suppress amyloid production. In the context of an IgM-related disorder, there is no therapeutic consensus, but it typically involves bendamustine and rituximab therapy followed by high-dose therapy and autologous stem cell rescue if fit.[53] Proteasome inhibitor–containing therapy should be used with caution in cases of neuropathy.[54]

Peripheral neurolymphomatosis in Waldenström macroglobulinemia. Cases caused by lymphoplasmacytic lymphoma (LPL) with IgM paraprotein are described.[55–57] LPL is a rare entity, and neuropathy can affect a combination of peripheral nerves, nerve roots, plexus, or cranial nerves. Invasion of the peripheral nervous system by LPL should come within the definition of Bing-Neel syndrome. Invasion can present with almost any of the aforementioned symptoms or signs; mono- or multiple neuropathies, confluent motor and sensory distal neuropathies, or proximal and distal weakness of a polyradiculoneuropathy reminiscent of chronic inflammatory demyelinating polyneuropathy (CIDP) can all be presenting features. Neuropathic pain is frequent. Cases progress over weeks and can be aggressive and disabling. Electrophysiology shows axonal neuropathy, sometimes with electrical "pseudoblock," which can also be confluent or patchy. Cerebrospinal fluid (CSF) can occasionally yield a diagnosis but frequently shows elevated protein, with or without pleocytosis. Cytological examination, immunophenotyping, and molecular studies, including polymerase chain reaction (PCR) for immunoglobulin heavy-chain variable-region (IgVH) rearrangements and *MYD88* mutations, are required to search for clonal cells. PET/computed tomography (CT) scans can sometimes identify affected nerves and may correlate with high-field MRI neurography images, with a higher diagnostic yield than with either modality alone. A nerve biopsy may be required, with a reported sensitivity of 30% to 100%.[55,58]

Other neuropathies
Chronic inflammatory demyelinating polyneuropathy. This type of neuropathy has been mentioned in several series but with few clinical details.[59,60] The prevalence of monoclonal gammopathy is 18% in idiopathic chronic inflammatory demyelinating polyneuropathy.[61] A demyelinating polyneuropathy in patients without anti-MAG antibodies may suggest a CIDP; despite the absence of an antibody, there is likely to be a causal link between IgM and neuropathy. The clinical picture of patients with demyelinating polyneuropathy is varied, with pure sensory, sensorimotor, or pure motor symptoms. A demyelinating neuropathy was the primary feature in three-quarters of the patients; early axonal loss during the neuropathy often leads to the suspicion of an associated hemopathy. Three main treatments are currently used: corticosteroids and IVIg as first-choice treatments and plasma exchange as an alternative.[37] In refractory or CIDP first-line–dependant patients, rituximab showed a 75% response rate and is effective in patients with an associated hematological disease.[62] The addition of alkylators, purine analogues, or steroids can be considered in refractory cases.[2]

Axonal neuropathies unrelated to the immunoglobulin M gammopathy. Patients with monoclonal IgM gammopathy may present with neuropathy due to another cause, such as diabetes, alcohol, or age. In the general population, in those older than 65 years, there is a prevalence of mild axonal slowly evolutive sensory neuropathy of 25%. In a prospective study, Levine and colleagues[60] found mild axonal sensory neuropathy to be the most frequent type of neuropathy in WM.

APPROACH TO DIAGNOSIS

The clinical history and examination are paramount to investigating a patient with suspected IgM-PN. Alternative causes of neuropathy should be considered, including hereditary neuropathies. Salient points in the clinical history, physical examination, and baseline investigations are outlined in **Table 1**. The Inflammatory Rasch-Built Overall Disability Scale (I-RODS) is the recommended disability assessment scale for inflammatory neuropathies, able to capture temporal changes in function.[63]

Table 1
Approach to diagnosis

History	Examination	Initial Investigations
Rate of progression	Peripheral nervous system	NCS and EMG
Clinical course—monophasic, relapsing and remitting, or progressing	Cranial nerve examination	B12 and folate, MMA, B9
Ataxia, falls	Fundoscopy	HbA1c
Motor vs sensory symptoms	Wasting	HIV antibody, hepatitis B core antibody, hepatitis B surface antigen, hepatitis C antibody, ± lyme serology
Tremor	Fasciculation	C3, C4 complement levels, ANA, and dsDNA
Atypical symptoms, including pain	Hepatosplenomegaly	Anti-MAG
Infective trigger	Macroglossia	Antiganglioside antibodies GQ1b, GM1, CD1a, GD1b, SGPG
Alcohol and drug exposure	Lying and standing blood pressure	+/− VEGF
Effect on functional abilities		Urine protein:creatinine ratio
Autonomic symptoms		Cryoglobulin testing (warmed tubes)
		NT-proBNP, troponin T
		+/TTR sequencing
		ECG
		Bone marrow aspirate morphology, immunophenotyping, MYD88L265P, trephine biopsy including Congo red staining
		CSF for cell count, protein, IgM, PCR for IgVH rearrangement and MYD88 mutations, immunophenotyping

Nerve Conduction Tests

Neurophysiologic examination, such as NCS and electromyography, is undertaken when PN is identified or suspected on clinical grounds; this determines the predominant targets of damage (conduction slowing and axonal), the pattern (sensory, motor, or sensorimotor and patchy or length dependent), and the extent of nerve damage.[2] Distinguishing between conduction slowing (demyelinating) and axonal neuropathy is essential to suggesting a pathomechanism, investigation, and eventual diagnosis of the neuropathy (**Figs. 1–3**).

Serological Testing

All patients with neuropathy and an IgM paraprotein should undergo testing for anti-MAG antibodies and a panel of antiganglioside antibodies, including anti-GM1 and the disialosyl gangliosides GD1b, GD3, GT1b, and GQ1b. A search for cryoglobulins with appropriate warmed tubes and transport chain, C3, C4 complement levels, ANA and dsDNA, glucose, free-light chain measurement, B12 and B9 vitamins, hepatitis and Lyme serologies and probably TTR sequencing should be considered in many. Cryoglobulinemia tests must be repeated before concluding their negativity.

Cerebrospinal Fluid Analysis

CSF analysis is indicated if there is clinical concern regarding direct lymphomatous central nervous system infiltration (Bing-Neel syndrome) or peripheral neurolymphomatosis. Traditional CSF analysis of total protein, glucose, and bacterial culture is inadequate in many patients. CSF proteins can be measured, including albumin, IgG, IgM, and beta-2 microglobulin, which is useful in determining CSF involvement. The CSF should also undergo a cellular count from a large sample and cytology. Immunophenotyping by flow cytometry and molecular studies, including PCR for IgVH rearrangement and *MYD88*[L265P] mutation in WM patients, are key investigations on CSF. Large-volume CSF (at least 5–10 mLs) and rapid examination (within hours) increase the diagnostic yield.[2] Immunophenotyping on a typical small-volume sample taken during a lumbar puncture or a long delay before the sample is processed leads to false-negative results.

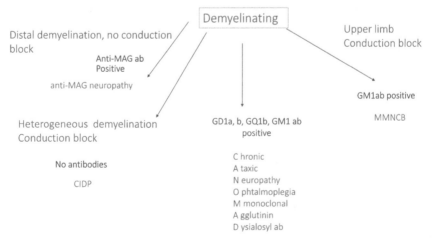

Fig. 1. Diagnostic algorithms of IgM-related neuropathy according to neurophysiological pattern. CIDP, chronic inflamatory demyelinating neuropathy; MMNCB, multifocal motor neuropathy with conduction block.

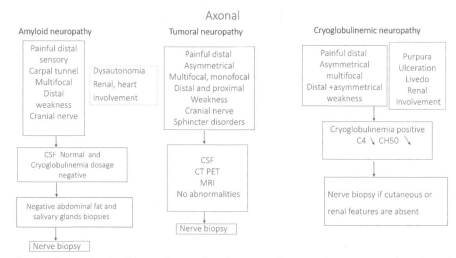

Fig. 2. Diagnostic algorithms of IgM-related neuropathy according to neurophysiological pattern.

Imaging

MRI must be performed before a lumbar puncture to avoid postprocedural spurious leptomeningeal enhancement, which could be misinterpreted as infiltrative disease. Targeted imaging should be obtained where there is suspicion of neural compression, leptomeningeal, or direct proximal radicular neural infiltration. The cauda equina has the best diagnostic yield. Imaging can assist in decisions regarding the optimal site of nerve biopsy but not the differential nature of nerve lesions.[2] Neurolymphomatosis is suggested if there is thickening and enhancement of individual nerves.[2,58] PET/CT scan has a higher diagnostic sensitivity than MRI alone for neurolymphomatosis and should be undertaken.[58,64]

Bone Marrow Aspirate and Trephine Biopsy

Most of the IgM-associated PN is caused by IgM MGUS.[65] Low-level MYD88-mutated small B-cell clones, identifiable only on flow cytometry on a bone marrow aspirate sample, have been identified in patients with an IgM-associated PN.[66] Indeed, the incidence of $MYD88^{L265P}$ may be higher in those with IgM paraproteins affected by neuropathy.[67] Compared with other patients with WM, those with PN have been found to have lower serum IgM and lower bone marrow disease burden,[7] perhaps a product of earlier diagnosis in the context of immune-mediated clinical symptoms prompting diagnostic evaluation. Bone marrow evaluation should be undertaken to demonstrate the nature of the underlying clonal disorder (immunophenotyping, PCR for $MYD88^{L265P}$), including evidence of these small clones, and has utility in suspected cases of AL amyloidosis, where a positive Congo red stain can prevent a sural nerve biopsy.

Nerve Biopsy

The role of nerve biopsy has diminished in recent years, as noninvasive diagnostic tests (such as anti-MAG antibody testing and CSF immunophenotyping) have facilitated nonbiopsy diagnosis. Nerve biopsy should be used in selected cases as a targeted diagnostic tool for neurolymphomatosis, amyloid, and vasculitis, synthetized

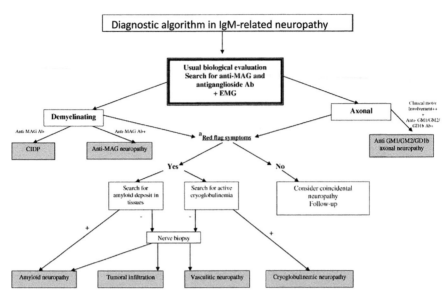

Fig. 3. Suggested strategy for diagnosing neuropathy in patients with Waldenström macroglobulinemia. [a]Red flag features are pain, multifocal topography, rapidly evolving course, cranial nerve involvement, dysautonomia, weight loss, cutaneous signs, heart/kidney/lung involvement, and abnormal serum-free light-chain concentration and ratio. Ab, antibodies; CIDP, chronic inflammatory demyelinating polyradiculoneuropathy; EMG, electromyography; MAG, myelin-associated glycoprotein. Usual biological evaluation including serum protein electrophoresis and immunofixation, free light chain in the serum, blood cell count, sedimentation rate, complement (hemolytic 50, C3, and C4 levels), rheumatoid factor, search for cryoglobulinemia, serum glucose, urea, and vitamin B12, Lyme, hepatitis, and HIV serologies. (*Adapted from* Viala K et al, 2012.)

in **Table 2**, guided by an experienced neurologist and hematologist and performed at a centre with expertise in peripheral nerve harvest and analysis.[2,68] Long-term sequelae, including pain and paraesthesia, are possible but infrequent, and thus the risks and benefits should be balanced.[2] Evidence of amyloid deposition should first be sought in other tissues, such as fat pad aspirate or trephine biopsy.

In cases of lymphocytic histological infiltration, immunophenotyping and molecular studies should be attempted to distinguish clonal from inflammatory infiltrate. Congo red staining for amyloid and kappa/lambda light chain immunostains can assist in clarifying pathology. Some stains and studies require an unfixed frozen nerve sample that must be determined before the biopsy, to be snap-frozen and not fixed.

TREATMENT SUMMARY

The presence of neuropathy alone is not an immediate indication for treatment, given the slowly progressive nature of the IgM-PN. To balance the risks and benefits of immunosuppressive treatments, a period of close monitoring is typically warranted initially, with documented progression prompting treatment.[2] Most of the clinical evidence is for anti-MAG PN, although even here, it is scant. Low-level MYD88-mutated small B-cell clones seem to be associated with treatment responsiveness to single-agent rituximab,[66] and a similar approach is taken to patients with underlying IgM MGUS. Patients with WM associated with a progressing IgM-PN are typically treated with

Table 2
Specific features of the individual immunoglobulin M peripheral neuropathies

Condition	Clinical	Electrophysiology	Antibody	Nerve Biopsy
Anti-MAG	• Slowly progressive distal sensory • Painless paraesthesia • Ataxia • Prominent tremor • Motor only in late	• Markedly prolonged distal latency index	MAG	Widened myelin lamellae
Multifocal motor neuropathy with conduction block	• Motor only • Distal, asymmetric upper limb weakness	Motor nerve conduction block as noncompressible sites	GM1/GD1b	May be normal
CANOMAD syndrome	• Distal sensory • Chronic ataxic neuropathy • Ophthalmoplegia +/− Bulbar palsies	Demyelinating pattern with very low or absent sensory action potentials and slow motor conduction velocities	GD1b/GD3/GT1b/GC1b	Demyelinating, axonal, and mixed features
Cryoglobulinemic vasculitis	• Painful distal sensory neuropathy with burning, shooting pains, and deep aching +/− Skin purpura +/− Renal involvement	Axonal length-dependent sensorimotor neuropathy often with an asymmetrical component	Negative	Large fiber degeneration, no regeneration, vasculitis, cryoglobulin deposition
AL amyloid	• Rapidly progressing sensorimotor • Painful, burning, allodynia • Autonomic symptoms	• May be normal Axonal sensorimotor neuropathy +/− median nerve entrapment • Abnormal thermal thresholds	Negative	Amyloid deposition on Congo red staining
Peripheral neurolymphomatosis	Mono- or multiple neuropathies, confluent motor and sensory distal neuropathies, or proximal and distal weakness of a polyradiculoneuropathy	Axonal neuropathy, sometimes with electrical "pseudoblock"	None	Lymphomatous infiltration

rituximab alone, dexamethasone-cyclophosphamide-rituximab, or bendamustine-rituximab. BTK inhibitors can also be considered according to local reimbursement arrangements.

SUMMARY

The IgM-PNs are a heterogeneous group of disorders capable of causing progressive patient disability. Although effective interventions can be used in patients with progressive symptoms, high-quality evidence is lacking, and disability may be irreversible. The collective experience of the peripheral nerve neurologist and hematologist in the clinic lies at the heart of early detection and timely intervention, alongside access to orthotics, specialist therapy services, and neuropathic adjuncts.

CLINICS CARE POINTS

- IgM is uniquely immunogenic but given the significant background rates of neuropathies and paraproteinaemia, their coexistence in an individual patient does not immediately infer causality.
- The various pathophysiologic mechanisms through which the underlying clonal disorder causes neuropathy determines different clinically distinct presentations.
- I-RODS is the recommended disability assessment scale for inflammatory neuropathies.
- Anti-MAG neuropathy represents half of the cases, with a classic clinical phenotype of progressive, symmetric distal sensory loss in the feet associated with early unsteadiness and frequently a complex tremor.
- The presence of neuropathy alone is not an immediate indication for treatment, given the slowly progressive nature of the IgM-peripheral neuropathies. To balance the risks and benefits of immunosuppressive treatments, a period of close monitoring is typically warranted initially, with documented progression prompting treatment.

DISCLOSURE

O. Tomkins, K. Viala, and D.R. Weil declare no conflicts of interests related to this publication. V. Leblond has received honoraria from Astra Zeneca, Abbvie, BeiGene, Janssen, Amgen Lilly, and MSD and is a consultant for Janssen, BeiGene, and Lilly. M.P. Lunn is PI for trials with Novartis and UCB Pharma; PI on Investigator led Optic, Perinoms, and IMAGiNe studies; DSMB for Octapharma trial and Investigator led IoC trial; has received honoraria from CSL Behring, Grifols, Novartis, UCB Pharma, and AstraZeneca pharmaceuticals; and ad hoc travel support grants from CSL Behring. S. D'Sa has received honoraria from BeiGene, Janssen, and Sanofi; was a consultant/advisor for Janssen, BeiGene, and Sanofi; received research funding from Janssen; and received travel and accommodations reimbursement from Janssen, BeiGene, and Sanofi.

REFERENCES

1. Tatum AH. Experimental paraprotein neuropathy, demyelination by passive transfer of human IgM anti-myelin-associated glycoprotein. Ann Neurol 1993;33(5):502–6.
2. D'Sa S, Kersten MJ, Castillo JJ, et al. Investigation and management of IgM and Waldenström-associated peripheral neuropathies: recommendations from the IWWM-8 consensus panel. Br J Haematol 2017;176(5):728–42.

3. Khwaja J, D'Sa S, Minnema MC, et al. IgM monoclonal gammopathies of clinical significance: diagnosis and management. Haematologica 2022;107(9):2037–50.
4. Notermans NC, Franssen H, Eurelings M, et al. Diagnostic criteria for demyelinating polyneuropathy associated with monoclonal gammopathy. Muscle Nerve 2000;23(1):73–9.
5. Kyle RA, Therneau TM, Rajkumar SV, et al. Prevalence of monoclonal gammopathy of undetermined significance. N Engl J Med 2006;354(13):1362–9.
6. Bardel B, Molinier-Frenkel V, Le Bras F, et al. Revisiting the spectrum of IgM-related neuropathies in a large cohort of IgM monoclonal gammopathy. J Neurol 2022;269(9):4955–60.
7. Treon SP, Hanzis CA, Ioakimidis LI, et al. Clinical characteristics and treatment outcome of disease-related peripheral neuropathy in Waldenstrom's macroglobulinemia (WM). J Clin Oncol 2010;28(15_suppl):8114.
8. Tomkins O, Lindsay J, Keddie S, et al. Neuropathy with IgM gammopathy: incidence, characteristics and management, a rory morrison W.M.U.K registry analysis. Blood 2020;136:1–2.
9. Nobile-Orazio E, Barbieri S, Baldini L, et al. Peripheral neuropathy in monoclonal gammopathy of undetermined significance: prevalence and immunopathogenetic studies. Acta Neurol Scand 1992;85(6):383–90.
10. Nobile-Orazio E, Meucci N, Baldini L, et al. Long-term prognosis of neuropathy associated with anti-MAG IgM M-proteins and its relationship to immune therapies. Brain 2000;123(4):710–7.
11. Svahn J, Petiot P, Antoine JC, et al. Anti-MAG antibodies in 202 patients: clinico-pathological and therapeutic features. J Neurol Neurosurg Psychiatr 2018;89(5):499–505.
12. Saifee TA, Schwingenschuh P, Reilly MM, et al. Tremor in inflammatory neuropathies. J Neurol Neurosurg Psychiatr 2013;84(11):1282–7.
13. Carroll AS, Lunn MPT. Paraproteinaemic neuropathy: MGUS and beyond. Practical Neurol 2021;21(6):492–503.
14. Kaku DA, England JD, Sumner AJ. Distal accentuation of conduction slowing in polyneuropathy associated with antibodies to myelin-associated glycoprotein and sulphated glucuronyl paragloboside. Brain 1994;117(5):941–7.
15. Takatsu M, Hays AP, Latov N, et al. Immunofluorescence study of patients with neuropathy and IgM M proteins. Ann Neurol 1985;18(2):173–81.
16. Yeung KB, Thomas PK, King RH, et al. The clinical spectrum of peripheral neuropathies associated with benign monoclonal IgM, IgG and IgA paraproteinaemia. Comparative clinical, immunological and nerve biopsy findings. J Neurol 1991;238(7):383–91.
17. European Federation of Neurological Societies/Peripheral Nerve Society Guideline on management of paraproteinemic demyelinating neuropathies. Report of a Joint Task Force of the European Federation of Neurological Societies and the Peripheral Nerve Society–first revision. J Peripher Nerv Syst 2010;15(3):185–95.
18. Nobile-Orazio E, Manfredini E, Carpo M, et al. Frequency and clinical correlates of anti-neural IgM antibodies in neuropathy associated with IgM monoclonal gammopathy. Ann Neurol 1994;36(3):416–24.
19. Chassande B, Léger J-M, Younes-Chennoufi AB, et al. Peripheral neuropathy associated with IgM monoclonal gammopathy: Correlations between M-protein antibody activity and clinical/electrophysiological features in 40 cases. Muscle Nerve 1998;21(1):55–62.

20. Vital A, Vital C, Julien J, et al. Polyneuropathy associated with IgM monoclonal gammopathy. Immunological and pathological study in 31 patients. Acta Neuropathol 1989;79(2):160–7.

21. Lunn MPT, Nobile-Orazio E. Immunotherapy for IgM anti-myelin-associated glycoprotein paraprotein-associated peripheral neuropathies. Cochrane Database Syst Rev 2016;10(10):CD002827.

22. Léger JM, Viala K, Nicolas G, et al. Placebo-controlled trial of rituximab in IgM anti-myelin-associated glycoprotein neuropathy. Neurology 2013;80(24): 2217–25.

23. Dalakas MC, Rakocevic G, Salajegheh M, et al. Placebo-controlled trial of rituximab in IgM anti-myelin-associated glycoprotein antibody demyelinating neuropathy. Ann Neurol 2009;65(3):286–93.

24. Steck AJ. Anti-MAG neuropathy: From biology to clinical management. J Neuroimmunol 2021;361:577725.

25. Nivet T, Baptiste A, Belin L, et al. Immunochemotherapy versus rituximab in anti-myelin-associated glycoprotein neuropathy: a report of 64 patients. Br J Haematol 2022;198(2):298–306.

26. Castellani F, Visentin A, Campagnolo M, et al. The Bruton tyrosine kinase inhibitor ibrutinib improves anti-MAG antibody polyneuropathy. Neurology - Neuroimmunology Neuroinflammation. 2020;7(4):e720.

27. Dimopoulos MA, Trotman J, Tedeschi A, et al. Ibrutinib for patients with rituximab-refractory Waldenström's macroglobulinaemia (iNNOVATE): an open-label substudy of an international, multicentre, phase 3 trial. Lancet Oncol 2017;18(2): 241–50.

28. Treon SP, Tripsas CK, Meid K, et al. Ibrutinib in previously treated Waldenström's macroglobulinemia. N Engl J Med 2015;372(15):1430–40.

29. Pestronk A, Cornblath DR, Ilyas AA, et al. A treatable multifocal motor neuropathy with antibodies to GM1 ganglioside. Ann Neurol 1988;24(1):73–8.

30. Galban-Horcajo F, Vlam L, Delmont E, et al. The diagnostic utility of determining anti-GM1: GalC complex antibodies in multifocal motor neuropathy: a validation study. J Neuromuscul Dis 2015;2(2):157–65.

31. Yeh WZ, Dyck PJ, van den Berg LH, et al. Multifocal motor neuropathy: controversies and priorities. J Neurol Neurosurg Psychiatr 2020;91(2):140–8.

32. van Schaik IN, van den Berg LH, de Haan R, et al. Intravenous immunoglobulin for multifocal motor neuropathy. Cochrane Database Syst Rev 2005;(2).

33. Van den Berg-Vos RM, Franssen H, Wokke JH, et al. Multifocal motor neuropathy: long-term clinical and electrophysiological assessment of intravenous immunoglobulin maintenance treatment. Brain 2002;125(Pt 8):1875–86.

34. Le Cann M, Bouhour F, Viala K, et al. CANOMAD: a neurological monoclonal gammopathy of clinical significance that benefits from B-cell–targeted therapies. Blood 2020;136(21):2428–36.

35. Willison HJ, O'Leary CP, Veitch J, et al. The clinical and laboratory features of chronic sensory ataxic neuropathy with anti-disialosyl IgM antibodies. Brain 2001;124(Pt 10):1968–77.

36. Yuki N, Uncini A. Acute and chronic ataxic neuropathies with disialosyl antibodies: a continuous clinical spectrum and a common pathophysiological mechanism. Muscle Nerve 2014;49(5):629–35.

37. Latov N. Diagnosis and treatment of chronic acquired demyelinating polyneuropathies. Nat Rev Neurol 2014;10(8):435–46.

38. Terrier B, Karras A, Kahn J-E, et al. The spectrum of type I cryoglobulinemia vasculitis: new insights based on 64 cases. Medicine 2013;92(2):61–8.

39. Terrier B, Krastinova E, Marie I, et al. Management of noninfectious mixed cryo-globulinemia vasculitis: data from 242 cases included in the CryoVas survey. Blood 2012;119(25):5996–6004.
40. Harel S, Mohr M, Jahn I, et al. Clinico-biological characteristics and treatment of type I monoclonal cryoglobulinaemia: a study of 64 cases. Br J Haematol 2015; 168(5):671–8.
41. Sidana S, Rajkumar SV, Dispenzieri A, et al. Clinical presentation and outcomes of patients with type 1 monoclonal cryoglobulinemia. Am J Hematol 2017;92(7): 668–73.
42. Néel A, Perrin F, Decaux O, et al. Long-term outcome of monoclonal (type 1) cry-oglobulinemia. Am J Hematol 2014;89(2):156–61.
43. Nemni R, Corbo M, Fazio R, et al. Cryoglobulinaemic neuropathy. A clinical, morphological and immunocytochemical study of 8 cases. Brain 1988;111(Pt 3):541–52.
44. Pouchelon C, Visentini M, Emmi G, et al. Management of nonviral mixed cryoglo-bulinemia vasculitis refractory to rituximab: data from a European collaborative study and review of the literature. Autoimmun Rev 2022;21(4):103034.
45. Gillmore JD, Wechalekar A, Bird J, et al. Guidelines on the diagnosis and inves-tigation of AL amyloidosis. Br J Haematol 2015;168(2):207–18.
46. Sachchithanantham S, Roussel M, Palladini G, et al. European collaborative study defining clinical profile outcomes and novel prognostic criteria in mono-clonal immunoglobulin M-related light chain amyloidosis. J Clin Oncol 2016; 34(17):2037–45.
47. Kapoor M, Rossor AM, Jaunmuktane Z, et al. Diagnosis of amyloid neuropathy. Practical Neurol 2019;19(3):250–8.
48. Viala K, Stojkovic T, Doncker A-V, et al. Heterogeneous spectrum of neuropathies in Waldenström's macroglobulinemia: a diagnostic strategy to optimize their man-agement. J Peripher Nerv Syst 2012;17(1):90–101.
49. Vital C, Vital A, Bouillot-Eimer S, et al. Amyloid neuropathy: a retrospective study of 35 peripheral nerve biopsies. J Peripher Nerv Syst 2004;9(4):232–41.
50. Gemignani F, Brindani F, Alfieri S, et al. Clinical spectrum of cryoglobulinaemic neuropathy. J Neurol Neurosurg Psychiatr 2005;76(10):1410–4.
51. Montcuquet A, Duchesne M, Roussellet O, et al. Electrochemical skin conduc-tance values suggest frequent subclinical autonomic involvement in patients with AL amyloidosis. Amyloid 2020;27(3):215–6.
52. Hazenberg BPC, Van Rijswijk MH, Piers DA, et al. Diagnostic performance of 123I-labeled serum amyloid P component scintigraphy in patients with amyloid-osis. Am J Med 2006;119(4):355, e15-e24.
53. Pratt G, El-Sharkawi D, Kothari J, et al. Diagnosis and management of Walden-ström macroglobulinaemia—A British Society for Haematology guideline. Br J Haematol 2022;197(2):171–87.
54. Wechalekar AD, Gillmore JD, Bird J, et al. Guidelines on the management of AL amyloidosis. Br J Haematol 2015;168(2):186–206.
55. Keddie S, Nagendran A, Cox T, et al. Peripheral nerve neurolymphomatosis: clin-ical features, treatment, and outcomes. Muscle Nerve 2020;62(5):617–25.
56. Ince PG, Shaw PJ, Fawcett PR, et al. Demyelinating neuropathy due to primary IgM kappa B cell lymphoma of peripheral nerve. Neurology 1987;37(7):1231–5.
57. Daher A, Kamiya-Matsuoka C, Woodman K. Patient With 2 Hematologic Malig-nancies Presenting as Neurolymphomatosis. J Clin Neuromuscul Dis 2018; 19(3):124–30.

58. Grisariu S, Avni B, Batchelor TT, et al. Neurolymphomatosis: an International Primary CNS Lymphoma Collaborative Group report. Blood 2010;115(24):5005–11.
59. Nobile-Orazio E, Marmiroli P, Baldini L, et al. Peripheral neuropathy in macroglobulinemia: Incidence and antigen–specificity of M proteins. Neurology 1987;37(9):1506–14.
60. Levine T, Pestronk A, Florence J, et al. Peripheral neuropathies in Waldenström's macroglobulinaemia. J Neurol Neurosurg Psychiatr 2006;77(2):224–8.
61. Maisonobe T, Chassande B, Vérin M, et al. Chronic dysimmune demyelinating polyneuropathy: a clinical and electrophysiological study of 93 patients. J Neurol Neurosurg Psychiatr 1996;61(1):36–42.
62. Roux T, Debs R, Maisonobe T, et al. Rituximab in chronic inflammatory demyelinating polyradiculoneuropathy with associated diseases. J Peripher Nerv Syst 2018;23(4):235–40.
63. Draak TH, Vanhoutte EK, van Nes SI, et al. Changing outcome in inflammatory neuropathies: Rasch-comparative responsiveness. Neurology 2014;83(23):2124–32.
64. Shaikh F, Chan AC, Awan O, et al. Diagnostic Yield of FDG-PET/CT, MRI, and CSF Cytology in Non-Biopsiable Neurolymphomatosis as a Heralding Sign of Recurrent Non-Hodgkin's Lymphoma. Cureus 2015;7(9):e319.
65. Sæmundur R, Vilhjálmur S, Ingemar T, et al. Peripheral neuropathy and monoclonal gammopathy of undetermined significance: a population-based study including 15,351 cases and 58,619 matched controls. Haematologica 2020;105(11):2679–81.
66. Chen LY, Keddie S, Lunn MP, et al. IgM paraprotein-associated peripheral neuropathy: small CD20-positive B-cell clones may predict a monoclonal gammopathy of neurological significance and rituximab responsiveness. Br J Haematol 2020;188(4):511–5.
67. Vos JM, Notermans NC, D'Sa S, Lunn MP, van der Pol WL, Kraan W, Reilly MM, Chalker J, Gupta R, Kersten MJ, Pals ST, Minnema MC. High prevalence of the MYD88 L265P mutation in IgM anti-MAG paraprotein-associated peripheral neuropathy. J Neurol Neurosurg Psychiatry 2018;89(9):1007–9.
68. Nathani D, Spies J, Barnett MH, et al. Nerve biopsy: Current indications and decision tools. Muscle Nerve 2021;64(2):125–39.

Evaluation and Management of Bing–Neel Syndrome

Sarah J. Schep, MD, PhD[a],*, Josephine M.I. Vos, MD, PhD[b],
Monique C. Minnema, MD, PhD[c]

KEYWORDS

- Bing–Neel syndrome • Waldenström macroglobulinemia • Central nervous system
- Cerebrospinal fluid • MRI

KEY POINTS

- Bing–Neel syndrome (BNS) is a rare manifestation of Waldenström macroglobulinemia (WM), which is caused by infiltration of lymphoplasmacytic lymphoma (LPL) cells in the central nervous system (CNS).
- Every WM patient with atypical or unexplained neurologic symptoms should be evaluated for BNS.
- Key in the diagnostic workup is an MRI of the brain and spine and cerebrospinal fluid (CSF) examination or (if possible) cerebral biopsy to confirm the presence of LPL cells in the CNS.
- Flow cytometry and molecular diagnostics aid in diagnosis by demonstrating a monoclonal B-cell population and the MYD88-mutation, respectively.
- The aim of the treatment is clinical improvement; BTK inhibitor ibrutinib is preferred as first-line therapy thanks to its high efficacy and limited toxicity.

INTRODUCTION

Bing–Neel syndrome (BNS) is an uncommon but serious manifestation of Waldenström macroglobulinemia (WM) caused by infiltration of the malignant lymphoplasmacytic cells in the central nervous system (CNS). The first report of this disorder dates to 1936, when the physicians Jens Bing and Axel Valdemar von Neel described two patients with hyperglobulinemia and subacute neurologic symptoms.[1] Remarkably, this was reported 8 years before Jan Waldenström described the disease we currently known as WM.[2] BNS represents an extramedullary presentation of WM, resulting in

[a] Department of Hematology, HAGA Ziekenhuis, Els Borst-Eilersplein 275, 2545 AA The Hague, The Netherlands; [b] Department of Hematology, Amsterdam UMC, University of Amsterdam, LYMMCARE, Cancer Center Amsterdam, Meibergdreef 9, Amsterdam & Sanquin, Meibergdreef 9, 1105 AZ Amsterdam, The Netherlands; [c] Department of Hematology, UMC Utrecht, Heidelberglaan 100, 3584 CX Utrecht, The Nehterlands
* Corresponding author.
E-mail address: s.schep@hagaziekenhuis.nl
Twitter: @MinnemaMonique (M.C.M.)

Hematol Oncol Clin N Am 37 (2023) 777–786
https://doi.org/10.1016/j.hoc.2023.04.008
0889-8588/23/© 2023 Elsevier Inc. All rights reserved.

a diverse spectrum of neurologic symptoms, ranging from headaches or gait disorders to cognitive deficits and psychiatric symptoms.[3,4] Given this clinical heterogeneity and rarity of the disorder, the recognition and early diagnosis of BNS are challenging. This review aims to summarize the current knowledge and guidelines regarding the clinical presentation, diagnosis, and treatment of BNS.

EPIDEMIOLOGY

The exact incidence of BNS is unknown but is estimated to occur in about 1% of WM cases.[5] WM itself is a rare lymphoid malignancy with an incidence of about three patients per million persons per year.[6] The disease is caused by an immunoglobulin M (IgM)-producing monoclonal lymphoplasmacytic infiltration in the bone marrow. The clinical picture of WM is very heterogeneous, ranging from asymptomatic to constitutional symptoms, complaints secondary to the IgM paraprotein (such as hyperviscosity or peripheral neuropathy), or anemia because of bone marrow infiltration. BNS is a rare manifestation of WM, affecting the cerebrospinal fluid (CSF), the meninges, and/or the brain parenchyma.

BNS can occur at any moment in the disease course of WM. The median time between the diagnosis of WM and BNS is 3 to 4 years, but in about 15% to 26% BNS represents the first manifestation of the disease.[3,4] The median age is 63 years, and BNS is more often seen in males. Remarkably, occurrence of BNS is independent of the systemic activity of WM. In about one-third of patients with BNS, the syndrome occurred while they received active treatment for WM, most of them also showing responsive disease or even complete remission.[4]

CLINICAL PRESENTATION

The clinical presentation of BNS is very diverse, and there are no pathognomonic symptoms for the disease. Together with the rarity of the disorder, this often results in a significant diagnostic delay. The median time between first symptoms and diagnosis of BNS is 4 months, whereas in about 20% of cases, the diagnosis was made after 1 year.[3]

The signs of BNS reflect the involvement of the CNS and are usually progressive over weeks to months (**Fig. 1**). Most described (30%–50%) symptoms are balance and gait disturbances, cranial nerve involvement (mainly oculomotor and facial nerves) and cognitive dysfunction such as confusion, memory loss, or altered mental status.[3,4,7] Headache or limb pain, sensory deficits or paresthesias, and seizures are seen in approximately 20% to 30% of patients.[3,4,7] Finally, visual abnormalities, hearing loss, and psychiatric symptoms can also occur in 10% to 20% of patients.[3,4,7]

It is important to discriminate between the signs of BNS and other comorbidities associated with WM, such as IgM-related polyneuropathy (PNP) or hyperviscosity syndrome. The most important differences between BNS and IgM-related PNP are summarized in **Table 1**. IgM-related PNP is characterized by a symmetrical pattern, affecting the distal nerves first. There is primarily sensory loss, and symptoms are slowly progressive over months to years. Moreover, anti-myelin-associated glycoprotein (MAG) antibodies can be identified in most cases. Contrary to this, sensorimotor symptoms in BNS show an asymmetric radicular distribution with a predominance of motor deficits. The disease course is more rapidly progressive over weeks to months.

Typical complaints associated with hyperviscosity are spontaneous nose bleeds, progressive headaches, and visual disturbances, such as blurry vision. Moreover, the high level of the serum IgM protein (symptomatic hyperviscosity is uncommon

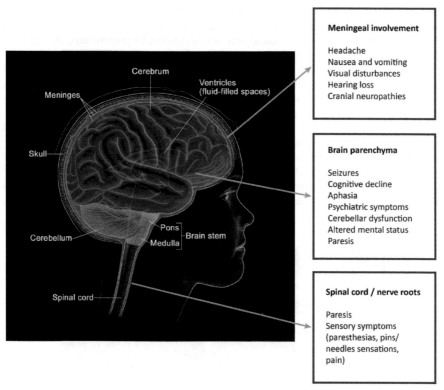

Meningeal involvement

Headache
Nausea and vomiting
Visual disturbances
Hearing loss
Cranial neuropathies

Brain parenchyma

Seizures
Cognitive decline
Aphasia
Psychiatric symptoms
Cerebellar dysfunction
Altered mental status
Paresis

Spinal cord / nerve roots

Paresis
Sensory symptoms
(paresthesias, pins/
needles sensations,
pain)

Fig. 1. Spectrum of clinical symptoms of Bing–Neel syndrome according to localization of CNS involvement.

with serum IgM levels <30 g/L) and typical findings by retinoscopy aid in differentiating between BNS and hyperviscosity syndrome.

DIAGNOSIS

Diagnosing BNS is challenging and requires a combination of clinical symptoms, blood and bone marrow examination, contrast-enhanced MRI of the brain and spine, and confirmation of the presence of lymphoplasmacytic lymphoma (LPL) cells in the CNS.

MRI of the brain and spinal cord is an important part of the diagnostic workup of BNS, both to support a diagnosis of BNS and exclude other causes and to identify

Table 1
Differences between immunoglobulin M-related polyneuropathy and Bing–Neel syndrome

	IgM PNP	Bing–Neel Syndrome
Pattern	Symmetrical Length-dependent (sock pattern) Mostly sensory loss	Asymmetrical Radicular distribution Mostly motor deficits
Disease course	Months to years	Weeks to months
Other	Anti-MAG positive EMG showing demyelination	

Abbreviations: Anti-MAG, anti-myelin associated glycoprotein; EMG, electromyography.

CNS tissue amenable to biopsy. MRI for fluid-attenuated inversion recovery (FLAIR) and T1-weighted sequences before and after gadolinium should be obtained to improve sensitivity. Moreover, radiological studies should be performed before lumbar puncture to prevent false-positive radiographic findings. The MRI abnormalities are seen in approximately 80% of patients; therefore, a normal scan does not rule out BNS.[3,4,8] In most cases (80%), MRI shows diffuse leptomeningeal enhancement, whereas in about 20%, tumoral masses are observed, usually located in periventricular/subependymal regions (**Fig. 2**).[8,9]

The demonstration of LPL cells in the CNS by biopsy of the cerebrum or meninges is the gold standard for diagnosing BNS.[10] In case a biopsy is not possible, a CSF examination to test the presence of LPL cells must be performed. In both cases, biopsy and CSF examination, transformation to a high-grade lymphoma must be excluded.[10]

When performing lumbar puncture for CSF examination, an adequate volume should be obtained for leucocyte count and differentiation, biochemical analysis,

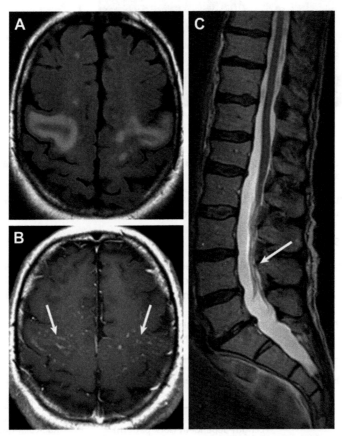

Fig. 2. MRI abnormalities in Bing–Neel syndrome. (*A*) Parenchymal involvement of the brain: Increased signal abnormalities in both precentral regions in axial FLAIR sequence. (*B*) Multiple nodular contrast enhancement in both precentral regions in axial T1 sequence after contrast media administration (see *arrows*). (*C*) Cauda equina thickening T2-sagittal sequence (see *arrow*). (Source (modified and re-used with permission): Minnema et al., Haematologica 2017.[10])

cytomorphology, flow cytometry, and molecular diagnostics.[10,11] The most frequent findings in the CSF are an elevated protein level and lymphocytic pleocytosis with cytomorphological atypical lymphocytes with a plasmacytic morphology (**Fig. 3**).[7] As these are all nonspecific findings, flow cytometry and molecular studies are essential in confirming BNS.

The role of flow cytometry is to demonstrate a clonal B-cell population. The flow cytometric profile of LPL is characterized by expression of the pan-B-cell markers CD19 and CD20, plasma cell markers CD138 and IgM, and restriction of the light chain.[12] Importantly, the immunophenotypic profile of the B-cell population in the CNS should be congruent with the malignant LPL cells in the bone marrow.

Molecular diagnostics detect Ig gene rearrangement or the presence of mutated MYD88 (L265P). Identifying a clonal relationship between Ig rearrangement of the LPL cells in the CNS and the bone marrow provides strong evidence supporting a diagnosis of BNS. The case series of Castillo and colleagues[4] demonstrated that an Ig rearrangement was observed in 94% of all cases. However, given the low cellular rate in the CSF, the sensitivity of this technique is limited. On the contrary, detection of the MYD88 L265P mutation by quantitative polymerase chain reaction (qPCR) is a very sensitive method and this mutation is seen in about 95% of all patients with BNS.[10] Given the high sensitivity of this method, caution must be taken to avoid blood contamination of the CSF to prevent false-positive results from LPL cells in the peripheral blood.[10] Blood contamination can be minimized by using the last diagnostic tube of CSF for this test. Finally, it should be noted that the MYD88-mutation is not specific to BNS, as it is also observed in primary CNS lymphoma (PCNSL) and rarely in other B-cell lymphomas.[13,14]

TREATMENT

Like WM, BNS is not curable, and treatment aims to improve the clinical symptoms and induce long progression-free survival.[10,11] Therapy is therefore only indicated in symptomatic patients with a definitive diagnosis of BNS. The complete eradication of all malignant cells in the CNS is not always possible and not necessary if patients have clinical benefit from the therapy similar to the treatment goals in WM and other indolent B-cell malignancies.

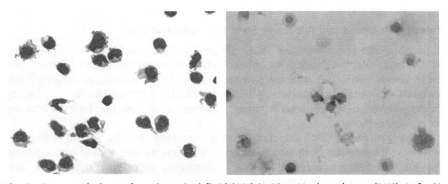

Fig. 3. Cytomorphology of cerebrospinal fluid (CSF) in Bing–Neel syndrome (BNS). Left: Giemsa stain of the CSF of a patient with BNS relapse after previous diagnosis of Waldenström macroglobulinemia. Right: kappa immunohistochemistry positivity of the lymphoplasmacytic lymphoma (LPL) cells, concordant with the LPL in bone marrow biopsy. (Source (reused with permission): Minnema et al., Haematologica 2017.[10])

As a result of the rarity of the disease, no randomized clinical trials have been performed and treatment advice is based on expert opinion and published case series. Earlier therapeutic options included chemotherapeutic agents with CNS penetration, intrathecal (IT) therapy, and radiotherapy (RT). The introduction of Bruton tyrosine kinase (BTK) inhibitors changed the treatment landscape of BNS (**Fig. 4**).[7,10,11]

Chemotherapy

Several chemotherapeutic options, with known or probable penetration of the blood–brain barrier, are suitable for treating BNS. Based on experiences treating PCNSL, one of the first therapies for BNS included high-dose methotrexate and high-dose cytarabine. Although effective, these treatments also carry high toxicity. Therefore, they should be reserved only for patients considered fit for intensive therapy. Other less toxic but effective treatment options include bendamustine or purine analogs such as fludarabine or cladribine.[15] Based on the two largest case series of BNS, the overall response rate of these agents was 70% with no differences between the various approaches.[3,4]

Bruton Tyrosine Kinase Inhibitors

The introduction of BTK inhibitors (BTKi) ibrutinib led to a breakthrough in treating BNS. After its demonstrated efficacy in WM, it was shown that ibrutinib penetrates the blood–brain barrier and is also effective in BNS.[16] Based on a retrospective case series of 28 patients, treatment with ibrutinib improved or resolved symptoms in 85% of patients.[17] Moreover, 83% had a decrease or resolution of radiologic abnormalities and in 47%, the disease was no longer detectable in the CSF.[17] The 2-year event-free survival was 80% and the 5-year survival rate 86%.[17] No differences were observed between the 420 and 560 mg doses and the toxicity was mild.[17]

Interesting in this regard is the introduction of the second-generation BTKi zanubrutinib, which bears higher selectivity for the BTK pathway and therefore has demonstrated fewer side effects. A randomized phase 3 trial in WM patients demonstrated that both zanubrutinib and ibrutinib are highly effective. Still, zanubrutinib was associated with less toxicity, particularly cardiovascular adverse events.[18] Experience with zanubrutinib in treating BNS is still limited, but the agent is already successfully used in a few cases.[19] Awaiting more results on the efficacy of zanubrutinib in BNS, it may have a role in treating BNS patients.

Role of Autologous and Allogeneic Stem Cell Transplantation

In patients with chemosensitive WM relapse, autologous stem cell transplantation (ASCT) is an effective therapeutic option.[20] Data regarding its role in BNS treatment are, however, limited. A retrospective case series by Simon and colleagues[20] describes 14 patients who underwent ASCT after induction treatment for BNS. The study cohort was very heterogeneous regarding treatment protocols used for induction and consolidation therapy.

In nearly all cases, BNS induction therapy consisted of systemic and IT therapy, often with the addition of rituximab. None of the patients was treated with ibrutinib. For the conditioning scheme, BEAM (carmustine, etoposide, cytarabine, and melphalan) or a thiotepa-based regimen was applied. All patients had chemosensitive disease before ASCT. With a median follow-up of 35 months, the overall response rate was 92% and only one patient relapsed. Five-year overall survival was 84%. Although these results of ASCT seem promising, the heterogeneity in treatment protocols (without incorporation of ibrutinib) and short follow-up make it difficult to determine

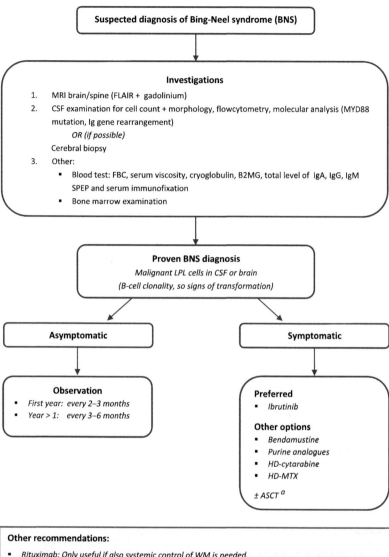

Fig. 4. Diagnostic workup and treatment of Bing–Neel syndrome (BNS). ASCT, autologous stem cell transplantation; B2MG, beta-2 microglobulin; CSF, cerebrospinal fluid; FBC, full blood count; FLAIR, fluid-attenuated inversion recovery; HD, high-dose; Ig, immunoglobulin; LPL, lymphoplasmacytic lymphoma; MTX, methotrexate; SPEP, serum protein electrophoresis. [a]ASCT can be considered in fit patients with relapsed disease showing chemosensitive disease. (Analogues to Minnema et al., Haematologica 2017, with permisson.[10])

the exact role and optimal timing for this relatively toxic treatment. It could, however, be considered in fit patients with relapsed disease.

To our knowledge, allogeneic stem cell transplantation (SCT) has not been used in BNS. In WM, the role of allogeneic SCT is very limited given the high non-relapse-associated mortality and the relatively low probability of long-term remission, rendering the newer, less toxic treatment options preferable.[21]

Other Treatment Options

Rituximab monotherapy is not recommended for treating BNS due to poor CNS penetration. Adding rituximab to other therapies, such as ibrutinib or chemotherapy, can be useful when systemic disease control is also needed. Experience with IT rituximab in BNS is limited. In other B-cell lymphomas involving the CNS, IT rituximab appeared effective but was also associated with serious toxicity. Therefore, its use is not advised as a first-line treatment.[22,23]

Other treatment options for BNS include IT chemotherapy and RT.[10,11] Monotherapy with IT drugs has been associated with short-lived responses. Therefore, if used, it is advised in combination with systemic therapy to treat meningeal involvement or in the palliative setting.

BNS is sensitive to RT, and effective use of RT is described in several case reports.[10,24] The downside of this therapeutic modality is the risk of neurotoxicity, especially the occurrence of late neurocognitive effects. For this reason, RT is not recommended as a first-line option but should be reserved for patients in the refractory of relapsed setting or in case of localized involvement of the CNS, such as exclusive cauda equina involvement in which toxicity is limited.[10,11]

TREATMENT OF OCULAR BING–NEEL SYNDROME

Although rare, involvement of the eye and surrounding structures may occur in BNS, requiring specific attention. Patients with new complaints of the eyes and/or sight should be evaluated by an ophthalmologist for an extended eye examination. A biopsy should be performed to confirm ocular involvement. For lesions in a surgically inaccessible site, conjunctival biopsy (or CSF examination) could be used as a surrogate.

Only a few cases of ocular BNS have been described in the literature and, in each case, a different treatment strategy was applied.[25–29] Most patients received a combination of intravenous (IV) and IT chemotherapy. In two of six patients, RT was also used. Treatment resulted in (at least) partial response in five patients, whereas one patient showed no improvement in vision despite aggressive treatment with IV high-dose methotrexate, IT cytarabine, and radiotherapy.[26]

PROGNOSIS

There are limited data on the prognosis of BNS and results are quite variable. The case series of Simon and colleagues[3] showed a 5-year survival rate of 71% and a 10-year survival rate of 59%, whereas in the cohort of Castillo and colleagues,[4] 3-year survival was 59%. For comparison, the median overall survival in WM is 9.2 years with a 10-year survival rate ranging from 84% in the very low-risk group to 9% in the very high-risk group.[30] The median progression-free survival after first-line treatment of BNS was 26 months.[3] Most deaths occur within 2 years of diagnosis, in 70% secondary to the progression of BNS or toxicity of treatment. There are no established prognostic factors, but no previous treatment for WM (3-year survival 100% vs 40%), age less than 65 years and platelet count greater than $100 \times 10^9/L$ all seem to be associated with a favorable prognosis.[4]

It should be noted that in the abovementioned studies, the treatment was heterogeneous, and the results predate the introduction of ibrutinib. Based on a retrospective case series, 5-year survival in patients treated with ibrutinib was 86%.[17] As such, it is expected that the prognosis of BNS nowadays might be more favorable than described above.

SUMMARY

All WM patients with unexplained neurologic symptoms must be evaluated for the presence of BNS to prevent diagnostic delay and the risk of permanent neurologic damage. Essential in the diagnostic workup is an MRI of the brain and spine and a CSF examination or cerebral biopsy to demonstrate the presence of LPL cells. As BNS is a non-curable disease, treatment should be aimed at improving symptoms. Several chemotherapeutic agents with good CNS penetration have proven efficacy in this syndrome. The introduction of ibrutinib has provided a breakthrough in treating BNS because of its high efficacy and is therefore preferred as the first-line therapy.

DISCLOSURE

S.J. Schep: nothing to disclose. M.C. Minnema: Speakers Bureau Janssen-Cilag, WebMD Global, Consultancy Janssen-Cilag, CDR-life, BMS, GSK, research funding; BeiGene; all honoraria are institutional. J.M.I. Vos: consultancy and advisory board (Sanofi), research funding (BeiGene, China & Abbvie, United States/Genmab), Speakers bureau and conference support (BMS); all honoraria are institutional.

REFERENCES

1. Bing J, von Neel A. Two cases of hyperglobulinaemia with affection of the central nervous system on a toxi-infectious basis. Acta Med Scand 1936;88:492–506.
2. Waldenström J. Incipient myelomatosis or essential hyperglobulinemia with fibrinogenopenia: a new syndrome? Acta Med Scand 1944;117:216–47.
3. Simon L, Fitsiori A, Lemal R, et al. Bing-Neel syndrome, a rare complication of waldenström macroglobulinemia: analysis of 44 cases and review of the literature. A study on behalf of the French Innovative Leukemia Organization (FILO). Haematologica 2015;100(12):1587–94.
4. Castillo JJ, D'Sa S, Lunn MP, et al. Central nervous system involvement by Waldenström macroglobulinaemia (Bing-Neel syndrome): a multi-institutional retrospective study. Br J Haematol 2016;172(5):709–15.
5. Kulkarni T, Treon S, Manning R, et al. Clinical characteristics and treatment outcome Of CNS involvement (Bing-Neel syndrome) in waldenstrom's macroglobulinemia. Blood 2013;122(21):5090.
6. Kyle RA, Larson DR, McPhail ED, et al. Fifty-year incidence of waldenström macroglobulinemia in olmsted county, minnesota, from 1961 through 2010: a population-based study with complete case capture and hematopathologic review. Mayo Clin Proc 2018;93(6):739–46.
7. Nanah A, al Hadidi S. Bing-neel syndrome: update on the diagnosis and treatment. Clin Lymphoma, Myeloma & Leukemia 2022;22(3):e213–9.
8. Fitsiori A, Fornecker LM, Simon L, et al. Imaging spectrum of Bing–Neel syndrome: how can a radiologist recognise this rare neurological complication of Waldenström's macroglobulinemia? Eur Radiol 2019;29(1):102–14.
9. Varettoni M, Defrancesco I, Diamanti L, et al. Bing-Neel syndrome: illustrative cases and comprehensive review of the literature. Mediterr J Hematol Infect Dis 2017;9(1):1–10.
10. Minnema MC, Kimby E, D'Sa S, et al. Guideline for the diagnosis, treatment and response criteria for Bing-Neel syndrome. Haematologica 2017;102(1):43–51.

11. Castillo JJ, Treon SP. How we manage Bing–Neel syndrome. Br J Haematol 2019; 187(3):277–85.
12. Owen R, Treon S, Al-Katib A, et al. Clinicopathological definition of Waldenstrom's macroglobulinemia: consensus panel recommendations from the Second International Workshop on Waldenstrom's Macroglobulinemia. Semin Oncol 2003; 30(2):110–5.
13. Ayanambakkam A, Ibrahimi S, Bilal K, et al. Extranodal marginal zone lymphoma of the central nervous system. Clin Lymphoma, Myeloma & Leukemia 2018;18(1):34–7.e8.
14. Yamada S, Ishida Y, Matsuno A, et al. Primary diffuse large B-cell lymphomas of central nervous system exhibit remarkably high prevalence of oncogenic MYD88 and CD79B mutations. Leuk Lymphoma 2015;56(7):2141–5.
15. Vos JMI, Kersten MJ, Kraan W, et al. Effective treatment of Bing-Neel Syndrome with oral fludarabine: a case series of four consecutive patients. Br J Haematol 2016;172(3):461–4.
16. Mason C, Savona S, Rini JN, et al. Ibrutinib penetrates the blood brain barrier and shows efficacy in the therapy of Bing Neel syndrome. Br J Haematol 2017;179(2): 339–41.
17. Castillo JJ, Itchaki G, Paludo J, et al. Ibrutinib for the treatment of Bing-Neel syndrome: a multicenter study. Blood 2019;133(4):299–305.
18. Tam CS, Opat S, D'Sa S, et al. A randomized phase 3 trial of zanubrutinib vs ibrutinib in symptomatic Waldenström macroglobulinemia: the ASPEN study. Blood 2020;136(18):2038–50.
19. Wong J, Cher L, Grif J, et al. Efficacy of zanubrutinib in the treatment of bing-neel syndrome. Hemasphere 2018;2(6):e155.
20. Simon L, Lemal R, Fornecker LM, et al. High-dose therapy with autologous stem cells transplantation in Bing-Neel syndrome: a retrospective analysis of 14 cases. Am J Hematol 2019;94(9):E227–9.
21. Chakraborty R, Muchtar E, Gertz MA. The role of stem cell transplantation in Waldenstrom's macroglobulinemia. Best Pract Res Clin Haematol 2016;29(2): 229–40.
22. Rubenstein JL, Fridlyand J, Abrey L, et al. Phase I study of intraventricular administration of rituximab in patients with recurrent CNS and intraocular lymphoma. J Clin Oncol 2007;25(11):1350–6.
23. Bromberg JEC, Doorduijn JK, Baars JW, et al. Acute painful lumbosacral paresthesia after intrathecal rituximab. J Neurol 2012;259(3):559–61.
24. Shimizu K, Fujisawa K, Yamamoto H, et al. Importance of central nervous system involvement by neoplastic cells in a patient with Waldenström's macroglobulinemia developing neurologic abnormalities. Acta Haematol 1993;90(4):206–8.
25. Stacy RC, Jakobiec FA, Hochberg FH, et al. Orbital involvement in bing-neel syndrome. J Neuro Ophthalmol 2010;30(3):255–9.
26. Doshi RR, Silkiss RZ, Imes RK. Orbital involvement in bing-neel syndrome. J Neuro Ophthalmol 2011;31:94–6.
27. Hughes MS, Atkins EJ, Cestari DM, et al. Isolated optic nerve, chiasm, and tract involvement in bing-neel syndrome. J Neuro Ophthalmol 2014;34(4):340–5.
28. Pham C, Griffiths JD, Kam A, et al. Bing-Neel syndrome – Bilateral cavernous sinus lymphoma causing visual failure. J Clin Neurosci 2017;45:134–5.
29. Gavriatopoulou M, Ntanasis-Stathopoulos I, Moulopoulos LA, et al. Treatment of bing-neel syndrome with first line sequential chemoimmunotherapy: a case report. Medicine 2019;98(44):e17794.
30. Kastritis E, Morel P, Duhamel A, et al. A revised international prognostic score system for Waldenström's macroglobulinemia. Leukemia 2019;33(11):2654–61.

Evaluation and Management of Disease Transformation in Waldenström Macroglobulinemia

Dipti Talaulikar, PhD, FRCPA, FRACP[a,b,]*, Cécile Tomowiak, MD[c],
Elise Toussaint, MD[d], Pierre Morel, MD[e],
Prashant Kapoor, MD, FACP[f], Jorge J. Castillo, MD[g],
Alain Delmer, MD[h], Eric Durot, MD[h]

KEYWORDS

- Diffuse large B-cell lymphoma • Waldenström macroglobulinemia
- Histologic transformation • $MYD88^{L265P}$ mutation

KEY POINTS

- Histologic transformation should be suspected in patients with WM that develop constitutional symptoms, rapidly progressive lymphadenopathy, extranodal involvement, sudden rise in LDH levels, and/or decreased serum IgM levels.
- Tissue biopsy is mandatory to diagnose histologic transformation and may be directed by clinical or radiologic features (ie, by site of rapidly enlarging lymph nodes, or by site of increased avidity on ^{18}FDG-PET/CT).
- Histologic diagnosis is required to confirm transformation to high-grade lymphoma. Most transformation events are caused by DLBCL variants, but rarely other aggressive lymphomas may occur.
- Treatment with intermediate-dose chemoimmunotherapy, such as R-CHOP, is the preferred option. CNS prophylaxis with HD-MTX should be considered if feasible and consolidation with autologous SCT should be discussed in fit patients responding to chemoimmunotherapy. If available, enrollment in clinical trials should be recommended.

[a] Department of Hematology, Canberra Health Services, Canberra, Australian Capital Territory, Australia; [b] College of Health and Medicine, Australian National University, Canberra, Australian Capital Territory, Australia; [c] Hematology Department and Centre d'Investigations Cliniques (CIC) 1082 INSERM, University Hospital, Poitiers, France; [d] Department of Hematology, Institut de Cancérologie Strasbourg Europe (ICANS), Strasbourg, France; [e] Department of Hematology, University Hospital of Amiens, Amiens, France; [f] Division of Hematology, Department of Internal Medicine, Mayo Clinic, Rochester, MN, USA; [g] Bing Center for Waldenström Macroglobulinemia, Dana-Farber Cancer Institute, Harvard Medical School, Boston, MA, USA; [h] Department of Hematology, University Hospital of Reims and UFR Médecine, Reims, France
* Corresponding author. Department of Hematology, Canberra Health Services, Canberra, Australian Capital Territory, Australia.
E-mail address: dipti.talaulikar@act.gov.au

Hematol Oncol Clin N Am 37 (2023) 787–799
https://doi.org/10.1016/j.hoc.2023.04.009

INTRODUCTION AND HISTORICAL PERSPECTIVES

Waldenström macroglobulinemia (WM) can undergo histologic transformation (HT) into aggressive lymphoma, usually diffuse large B-cell lymphoma (DLBCL) of the activated B-cell (ABC) subtype.

This phenomenon was first reported by Wood and Frenkel[1] in 1967 in a patient with WM who developed multiple lymphoblastic lymphosarcomatous masses. Initial case reports described HT in WM as "reticulum cell sarcoma" or "immunoblastic sarcoma."[2-6] A case series of 16 patients highlighted common features, such as rapid growth of lymph nodes, physical deterioration, decrease in serum monoclonal IgM level, and a poor prognosis with a median survival of 2 months.[7]

More recent retrospective studies have reported survival of approximately 1.5 to 2.7 years with chemoimmunotherapy (CIT).[8-10] Patients with HT often present with high rates of extranodal involvement and high International Prognostic Index (IPI) scores. The importance of MYD88 status in conferring risk for HT and as a prognostic factor after HT has been reported in multiple studies.[10-12] CIT treatments used in de novo DLBCL are less successful in HT with reported median survival after HT of 16 months to 2.7 years,[10,11] resulting from refractory disease or relapse, and a high frequency of central nervous system (CNS) involvement.[11,13] Clinical trials are difficult to conduct in such a rare disease; however, novel agents may be trialed in these patients. The role of stem cell transplantation (SCT) is not established.

DISCUSSION
Epidemiology and Risk Factors

HT to aggressive B-cell lymphoma is estimated to occur in 1% to 4% of patients with WM.[9,10] Two large centers in the United States have reported 5-, 10-, and 15-year cumulative incidence rates of transformation of 1%, 2%, and 4%; and 2%, 5%, and 6%. The 6-year cumulative incidence of HT was reported to be 8% in the fludarabine arm and 11% in the chlorambucil arm in the randomized WM1 trial, which compared fludarabine and chlorambucil.[14] The median time to transformation is reported to be 4.3 to 4.6 years.[8-11] About 15% to 25% of patients are reported to be treatment-naive at the time of HT.[8-10]

The high rate of HT in patients treated with nucleoside analogues found in some retrospective studies[15] has not been confirmed in the randomized WM1 trial.[14] The risk of HT in patients treated with Bruton tyrosine kinase (BTK) inhibitors is unknown.[16-19]

Data on risk factors for development of HT in WM are sparse. The $MYD88^{WT}$ genotype has been shown to be independently associated with a higher risk of HT.[10,12] HT occurred in 15% of $MYD88^{WT}$ compared with only 1% in $MYD88^{L265P}$ mutated patients, with a 10-year cumulative incidence of 20% and 1%, respectively.[12] Another study reported that $MYD88^{WT}$ was associated with a shorter time to HT (hazard ratio, 7.9; $P = 0.001$) (**Fig. 1**); furthermore, it was the only factor associated with an increased risk of HT in a multivariate analysis (odds ratio, 7; $P = 0.003$).[10] There are several mutations reported in $MYD88^{WT}$ patients affecting nuclear factor-κB signaling (TBL1XR1, NFKBIB, NFKBIZ, NFKB2, MALT1, BCL10), DNA damage repair (TP53, ATM, and TRRAP), and epigenomic regulators (KMT2D, KMT2C, and KDM6A), many of which are also reported in DLBCL; these are hypothesized to contribute to the increased risk of HT.[20]

Clinical Features

Patients with WM who develop rapidly enlarging lymphadenopathy, progressive constitutional symptoms, physical decline, rise in serum lactate dehydrogenase (LDH) levels, and/or extranodal involvement should be suspected to have HT. Most

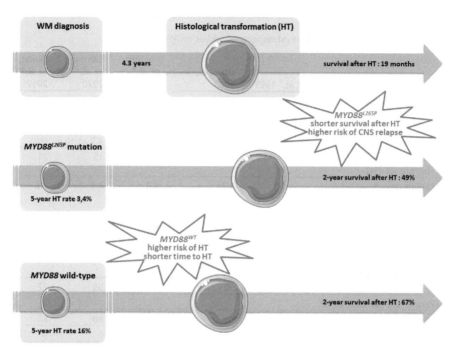

Fig. 1. Schematic representation of HT in WM. Transformation rates, time to HT, and survival after HT according to *MYD88* status. (*From* Durot et al.[65])

patients with HT present with advanced Ann Arbor stage disease and high IPI score. Transformed WM is often associated with a decrease in serum IgM levels.[8,10] This may be because of HT developing while patients are responding to treatment of underlying WM and/or be related to a process of dedifferentiation. Extranodal involvement, which is rare in WM (4.4%), is a common feature in HT, and is reported to occur in 70% to 90% of patients (**Table 1**).[8–10,21] Although skeletal bone and bone marrow are the most common sites of involvement, there is a high frequency of CNS, testis, and skin involvement.[8,13,22] The de novo DLBCL counterpart of transformed *MYD88*-associated sites (CNS, testis) is now a distinct entity, called "large B-cell lymphomas of immune-privileged sites" in the recent World Health Organization Classification of hematolymphoid tumors.[23] It includes aggressive tumors of ABC phenotype, characterized by concomitant *MYD88* and *CD79B* mutations and poor prognosis.[24]

Diagnosis

Histologic confirmation of high-grade lymphoma with a tissue biopsy is the gold standard to diagnose HT. The choice of the site of biopsy may be directed by clinical features (ie, site of rapidly increasing lymphadenopathy), or preferably, by high maximum standardized uptake value (SUVmax) on ^{18}fluorodeoxyglucose-PET/computed tomography (^{18}FDG-PET/CT).[8,25] The median SUVmax in a study of 24 transformed patients with WM was 15 (range, 4–38) and 71% presented with an SUVmax greater than 10[8], contrasting with 35 patients with nontransformed WM, in which 77% had positivity on ^{18}FDG-PET/CT with a mean SUVmax of 3 (range, 1–8).[26] Further studies are needed in WM to evaluate positive and negative predictive values of ^{18}FDG-PET/CT in HT diagnosis.

Table 1
Summary of the main published retrospective studies on HT in WM

Study	Garcia et al,[1] 1993	Lin et al,[27] 2003	Castillo et al,[9] 2016	Zanwar et al,[10] 2020	Durot et al,[8] 2017
Number of patients	16 (including 14 from literature review)	12	20	50	77
Incidence of HT (%)	NA	13	2.4 at 10 y	4.7 at 10 y	NA
Treatment naive before HT (%)	7	25	25	15	21
Median time from WM diagnosis to HT (y)	4	3.7	4.4	4.5	4.6
Male sex (%)	69	33	60	66	65
Median age at HT	NA	68	70	66	71
Extranodal involvement (%)	NA	100	84	72	91
Elevated LDH (%)	NA	80	67	53	72
Front-line treatment of HT					
R-CHOP-like (%)	NA	33	80	80	85
HyperCVAD (%)	NA	58	0	0	0
Rituximab-containing regimen (%)	NA	42	85	69	83
Autologous SCT (%)	NA	8	30	NA	15
Overall response rate (%)	NA	NA	NA	73	61
Complete response (%)	NA	NA	77	53	48
Progression-free survival (mo)	NA	NA	NA	10	9
Survival after HT (mo)	2	75 died within 10 mo	32	38	16

Abbreviations: CVAD, cyclophosphamide, vincristine, doxorubicin, and dexamethasone; NA, not available; R-CHOP, rituximab, cyclophosphamide, doxorubicin, vincristine, and prednisone.
From Durot et al.[65]

Histology

Although most transformation events are associated with the emergence of DLBCL variants,[8–10,27] cases of anaplastic large-cell lymphoma, T-cell lymphoma, plasma cell proliferation and Epstein-Barr virus-associated DLBCL, lymphomas intermediate between DLBCL and Burkitt lymphoma, or aggressive lymphomas, not otherwise specified have also been described.[28]

The histologic appearance of DLBCL is characterized by large B cells with frequent mitotic figures, resembling centroblasts (75% of cases) or immunoblasts (25% of cases).[27] Ki67 is high with a positive expression in 80% to 90% of the malignant cells.[8,9] Using the Hans algorithm,[29] about 80% to 90% of cases are classified as non-germinal center B-cell subtype.[8,10] CD20 is positive in 95% of patients using immuno-histochemistry, CD10 in 7% to 10%, BCL6 in 34% to 78%, MUM1 in 78% to 100%,

BCL2 in 86% to 89%, and MYC in 44% to 7%.[8–10] Most transformed WM (83%–100%) are negative for Epstein-Barr virus-encoded RNA in situ hybridization.[8–10,27] *MYC* gene rearrangement is seen in 11% to 38% of patients by fluorescence in situ hybridization,[8,10] but cases with *MYC* and *BCL2* and/or *BCL6* rearrangements ("double-hit" or "triple-hit" lymphomas) are not seen; a series of seven cases reported no cases that were found using fluorescence in situ hybridization.[30]

Biology and Clonal Evolution

Most (80%) high-grade transformation (ie, Richter syndrome) in chronic lymphocytic leukemia are clonally related to the underlying indolent condition.[31] In transformed WM, analysis of light-chain expression is reported to be similar in WM and transformed lymphoma cells in 75% to 100% of cases.[8,10] Using $MYD88^{L265P}$ mutation and immunoglobulin gene heavy chain variable region analysis, an Australian study on four cases of transformed and paired antecedent WM samples showed that DLBCL can be clonally related to WM or occur as a new clone independent of WM (synchronous de novo DLBCL).[32] More recently, MYD88L265P mutation, immunoglobulin gene heavy chain variable region rearrangement analyses, and next-generation sequencing were reported in seven patients who presented with lymphoplasmacytic lymphoma and DLBCL, with DLBCL being the first malignancy in some cases.[30] Three mechanisms of DLBCL development have been proposed: (1) "true" transformation with sequential mutation acquisition from WM to DLBCL, (2) clonal identity with a common origin but divergent evolution of WM and DLBCL, and (3) different lymphomas. A branching model of evolution has also been described with a transformed clone that did not evolve from the same subclone responsible for progression.[33]

There is limited understanding of the biology of transformation of WM to DLBCL. Whole-exome sequencing in four patients with WM who transformed to DLBCL showed genetic heterogeneity and complexity.[33] HT is associated with a much higher frequency of mutations and time of transformation is inversely related to mutation burden. Possible driver mutations within a high proportion of tumor cells that are conserved during transformation are identified. Additional and recurrent mutations are gained at HT including *PIM1*, *FRYL*, *PER3*, *PTPRD*, and *HNF1B*. *CD79B* mutations are postulated to be biomarkers predicting HT, being found mutated in three of the four evaluated cases.[33]

Prognosis

The outcome of patients with transformed WM is generally poor with overall survival (OS) after HT reported to vary from 16 to 38 months (see **Table 1**).[8–11] Zanwar and colleagues[10] reported a hazard ratio of 5.1 for death (95% confidence interval, 3.8–6.8; $P < 0.001$) and Castillo and colleagues[9] reported a much shorter median OS from diagnosis of WM to all-cause death of 9 versus 16 years for HT and non-HT patients.

Durot and colleagues,[8] in their cohort of 77 patients with transformed WM, showed that two or more lines of treatment of WM, prior rituximab exposure, time to transformation 5 or more years from WM diagnosis, elevated serum LDH, and less than partial response (PR) to DLBCL treatment were associated with shorter OS after transformation in univariate analysis. Time to transformation 5 or more years and elevated serum LDH retained significance in multivariate analysis. Longer time to transformation is also reported to adversely affect prognosis in Richter syndrome,[34] and outcome in transformed follicular lymphoma is worsened by previous therapy[35]; but there are conflicting data on the prognostic value of time to transformation in follicular lymphoma.[35,36] Concurrent diagnosis of indolent lymphoma and DLBCL has been reported to be associated with comparable outcomes to de novo DLBCL.[37] However, because there were only two cases of transformed lymphoplasmacytic lymphoma in the cohort and no cases of transformed WM, there are no data on how prognosis of HT in WM compares with DLBCL.[37]

The best evidence on prognosis in WM with HT comes from an international collaborative study in the form of a validated prognostic index, called the transformed Waldenström International Prognostic Index (tWIPI).[11] A training cohort of 133 patients was used to develop the index; three variables including high serum LDH (scored with 2 points), platelet count less than 100×10^9/L, and previous treatment of WM (both scored with 1 point each) were noted to be independently predictive of 2-year survival after HT. Three risk groups were defined: low-risk (0–1 point; 24% of patients), intermediate-risk (2–3 points; 59%), and high-risk (4 points; 17%), with 2-year survival rates of 81%, 47%, and 21%, respectively. This model was validated in an independent cohort of 67 patients and displayed high discrimination and calibration properties (Harrell C-index of 0.75 in the training cohort and 0.79 in the validation cohort).

In Richter syndrome, patients with clonally unrelated DLBCL, which accounts for 20% of cases, experience longer survival, comparable with patients with de novo DLBCL.[31] The clonal relationship between WM and DLBCL was not reported in the largest retrospective studies that analyzed clinical outcomes, precluding any conclusion of potential prognostic value of clonal relationship in transformed WM.[8–11]

MYD88 mutation status at time of WM seems to have a prognostic impact on survival after HT (see **Fig. 1**).[11] In the tWIPI study, *MYD88* mutation status was known in 64 patients. Patients with $MYD88^{L265P}$ mutation had a significantly lower 2-year survival rate after HT compared with patients with $MYD88^{WT}$ disease (49% vs 67%; $P = 0.018$). This finding, which is consistent with previous studies in de novo DLBCL,[38,39] requires confirmation in a larger cohort. The presence of $MYD88^{L265P}$ mutation has also been associated with a higher incidence of CNS relapse in transformed WM (17% vs 0% for $MYD88^{WT}$ patients).[13] In this study, the median survival after CNS relapse was 6 months.

Treatment Options

Given the rarity of the disease, there have been no prospective trials in transformed WM. Patients with transformed WM are usually excluded from clinical trials or represent a minority of patients among transformed indolent lymphomas. The recommendations on the treatment of transformed WM are therefore drawn from retrospective studies and from transformation of other indolent lymphomas. It should be kept in mind that patients can also be treated with palliative intent, reflecting the underlying comorbidities and frailty of this population.

Chemotherapy

Treatment of transformed WM usually mirrors DLBCL and involves use of CIT. Data on response rates and outcomes are based on retrospective studies. The most frequent frontline regimen used in HT is R-CHOP (rituximab, cyclophosphamide, doxorubicin, vincristine, and prednisone)-like CIT, which has been reported in 62% to 85% of cases, with overall response rates of 61% to 79%, complete response (CR) rates of 48% to 77%, and short median progression-free survival of 7 to 10 months (see **Table 1**).[8,10]

Data on more aggressive CIT regimens, such as R-EPOCH (rituximab, etoposide, prednisone, vincristine, cyclophosphamide, and doxorubicin) or ACVBP (doxorubicin, cyclophosphamide, vinblastine, bleomycin, and prednisone), are limited. In the study by Lin and colleagues,[27] 7 of 12 patients were treated with hyper-CVAD (fractioned cyclophosphamide, vincristine, doxorubicin, and dexamethasone), of which six died within the first 5 months; one patient was alive at 8 months after consolidation with BEAM (carmustine, etoposide, cytarabine, and melphalan) and autologous SCT (autoSCT). Other therapies used in frontline setting are DHAP (dexamethasone, cytarabine, and cisplatin), ICE (ifosfamide, cyclophosphamide, and etoposide), and GEMOX (gemcitabine and oxaliplatin).[8]

Autologous stem cell transplantation

High-dose chemotherapy consolidation followed by autoSCT in first CR (CR1) can be considered in fit patients with transformed indolent lymphomas, because of the poor prognosis associated with HT; however, it should be recognized that this is not based on strong evidence.[40–45] The retrospective studies available in transformed indolent lymphoma are mainly in transformed follicular lymphoma and have heterogeneous populations including patients in first or later remission and variable treatment regimens.[41–45] There are few WM patients with HT in these reports. There have been two case reports of transformed WM treated with allogeneic SCT[40] and only one WM case in a recent study of 49 patients investigating autoSCT in first remission.[46]

In the setting of transformed WM, a study reported one patient treated with hyper-CVAD followed by BEAM (carmustine, etoposide, cytarabine, and melphalan) conditioning and autoSCT.[27] In another cohort, 6 out of 20 patients received autoSCT with no survival benefit ($P = 0.13$).[9] This may be partly related to the fact that five patients underwent autoSCT at HT relapse and only one while in CR1. Another study did not find survival benefit in patients who underwent autoSCT ($P = 0.4$); however, only a few patients (3 out of 50) received it as consolidation after frontline therapy.[10] Ten (13%) of 77 patients underwent autoSCT, including seven after first-line treatment of HT in another series,[8] with a plateau emerging with use of autoSCT in patients responsive to frontline therapy (median OS not reached vs 4.5 years for responding non-autoSCT patients), although this was not statistically significant ($P = 0.33$).

Given that a randomized trial to elucidate the role of autoSCT in transformed WM is not likely to be feasible because of the rarity of the diagnosis, the role of consolidative autoSCT as part of frontline therapy for transformed WM in eligible patients remains unclear. Nevertheless, most patients with transformed WM are unfit (because of age or comorbidities) or do not achieve adequate response to proceed to autoSCT.

Central nervous system prophylaxis

Relapse within the CNS occurs in 2% to 5% of DLBCL cases and is associated with poor prognosis with median OS of 5 to 6 months.[47–49] The incidence of CNS relapse in transformed WM has been recently reported, with a 3-year rate of 11%, which is similar to that observed in the CNS-IPI high-risk group.[13,47] Patients with kidney/adrenal involvement and/or $MYD88^{L265P}$ mutation have a higher incidence of CNS relapse. Optimal CNS prophylaxis in these situations remains unknown because there is some evidence that intrathecal therapy is ineffective[50] and recent studies have reported lack of benefit with high-dose methotrexate (HD-MTX).[51,52] If HD-MTX is considered, recent studies in DLBCL suggest its delivery could be deferred beyond cycle 1 of R-CHOP (on Day 1 and especially before Day 10) or even until R-CHOP completion to avoid toxicities and/or R-CHOP delays.[53,54]

Novel agents

BTK inhibitors,[16–19] and BCL2 inhibitors, such as venetoclax,[55] show efficacy in WM and likely represent potential therapeutic options in transformed WM, given that expression of BCL2 is seen in 90%, and $MYD88^{L265P}$ mutation in 67% of cases. R-CHOP with concomitant ibrutinib showed improvement in event-free survival, progression-free survival, and OS in patients aged less than 60 years in a phase 3 study in ABC DLBCL.[56] However, patients older than 60 years showed increased toxicity with this regimen. Efficacy and safety of venetoclax associated with R-CHOP in the phase 2 CAVALLI study showed increased myelosuppression and potentially improved outcomes in BCL2+ subgroups.[57]

Chimeric antigen receptor T cells

CD19-targeted chimeric antigen receptor (CAR) T-cell therapies can lead to durable responses in relapsed/refractory (R/R) DLBCL, including transformed follicular lymphomas.[58,59] These therapies were initially used in third-line treatment of R/R DLBCL; however, their role as second-line treatment has now been established.[60,61] In R/R WM, efficacy of CD19-directed CAR T-cell therapy has been reported in three heavily pretreated patients, none of whom had transformed WM.[62] Abramson and colleagues[63] described use of lisocabtagene maraleucel in DLBCL transformed from indolent lymphoma. Eighteen patients had nonfollicular transformed indolent lymphomas, including two transformed WM; however, individualized data were not available from the study.[63] The potential effectiveness of CAR T-cell therapy in R/R transformed WM has recently been demonstrated in a case report of a 71-year-old man who received two prior lines of treatment of WM before HT. R-CHOP in

Table 2
Key points on clinical presentation, diagnosis, prognosis, and treatment of HT in WM

Clinical presentation	High frequency of extranodal involvement, in particular skeletal bone, bone marrow, and *MYD88*-associated sites (CNS, testis, skin)
	Advanced stage and high IPI score
	Elevated LDH
	Decrease in serum IgM spike
Diagnosis	Suspect HT in case of physical deterioration in patients with WM, rapid growth of lymph nodes, extranodal involvement, and/or rise in LDH level
	Tissue biopsy required for diagnosis of HT
	Tissue biopsy may be directed by [18]FDG-PET/CT
Prognosis	Poor outcome after HT
	Prognosis index (tWIPI) based on 3 predictors of 2-y survival after HT: elevated LDH (2 points), platelet count $<100 \times 10^9$/L (1 point), and any previous treatment of WM (1 point)
	Presence of *MYD88^{L265P}* mutation: lower 2-y survival after HT and higher risk of CNS relapse
Treatment	Treatment with similar regimens used in de novo DLBCL (R-CHOP-like regimen)
	ORR 61%–79%
	CR 48%–77%
	PFS 7–10 mo
	Insufficient data on more aggressive chemoimmunotherapy regimens
	Use of second-line chemoimmunotherapy regimens, such as RICE, are reasonable options for those rare patients that may have received anthracyclines for WM
	CNS prophylaxis should be considered (HD-MTX)
	Autologous SCT as consolidation in fit patients responding to induction chemotherapy should be considered
	Insufficient data on allogeneic SCT, novel agents, CAR T cells

Abbreviations: CAR, CD19-targeted chimeric antigen receptor; CR, complete response; [18]FDG-PET/CT, [18]fluorodeoxyglucose-PET/computed tomography; HD-MTX, high-dose methotrexate; ORR, overall response rate; PFS, progression-free survival; tWIPI, transformed Waldenström International Prognostic Index.
From Durot et al.[65]

combination with ibrutinib was used at HT. He then failed R-DHAP + autoSCT and was treated with axicabtagene ciloleucel following cytoreduction with fludarabine and cyclophosphamide, which induced CR on PET/CT and bone marrow biopsy, which was maintained at 1 year.[64] More data on use of this therapy for HT are needed.

SUMMARY

This paper details the clinical presentation, diagnosis, prognosis and treatment of histological transformation in WM (**Table 2**). The outcome of patients with transformed WM in retrospective studies remains poor. Whether increasing use of novel agents, such as BTK inhibitors or CAR T-cell therapy in WM, will change the frequency and outcomes of HT in WM remains unknown.

A deeper understanding of the biology and the pathophysiology of the disease, and prospective studies using novel therapies, are needed to improve clinical outcomes. This is particularly relevant for elderly, frail patients who are not fit for intermediate-dose CIT and stem cell transplant. International collaborations are required to deepen the understanding of this rare condition.

CLINICS CARE POINTS: RECOMMENDATIONS FOR MANAGEMENT OF HISTOLOGIC TRANSFORMATION IN WALDENSTRÖM MACROGLOBULINEMIA

Recommendations for optimal management of HT in WM are limited by the lack of prospective data and are therefore drawn from retrospective studies.

- HT should be suspected in patients with WM that develop constitutional symptoms, rapidly progressive lymphadenopathy, extranodal involvement, sudden rise in LDH levels, and/or decreased serum IgM levels.

- Tissue biopsy is mandatory to diagnose HT and may be directed by clinical or radiologic features (ie, by site of rapidly enlarging lymph nodes, or by site of increased avidity on [18]FDG-PET/CT).

- Histologic diagnosis is required to confirm transformation to high-grade lymphoma. Most transformation events are associated with the emergence of DLBCL variants, but other aggressive lymphomas may occur rarely.

- Treatment with intermediate-dose CIT, such as R-CHOP, is the preferred option. CNS prophylaxis with HD-MTX should be considered if feasible and consolidation with autologous SCT should be discussed in fit patients responding to CIT. If available, enrollment in clinical trials should be recommended.

AUTHORSHIP

Dr. Talaulikar receives research funding from Roche, Takeda and Janssen, honoraria from Janssen, Roche, Beigene, Takeda, Antengene, EUSA and CSL. Dr. Tomawiak receives research funds from Gilead and Roche, honoraria from Abbvie, Janssen, Beigene and AstraZeneca. Dr. Toussaint receives no diclosures. Dr. Morel receives honoraria from Beigene, AstraZeneca and Janssen. Dr. Kapoor receives research funding Amgen, Regeneron, BMS, LOXO, Ichnos, Karyopharm, Sanofi, Abbvie, GSK. Consultancy/advisory boards of Beigene, Pharmacyclics, X4 pharmaceuticals, Oncopeptides, Angitia Bio, GSK, AbbVie and Sanofi. Dr. Castillo receives research funds from Abbvie, AstraZeneca, Beigene, Cellectar, LOXO, Pharmacyclics, TG Therapeutics. Honoraria from Abbvie, Beigene, Cellectar, Kite, LOXO, Janssen, Pharmacyclics and Roche. Drs. Delmer and Durot: no disclosures.

REFERENCES

1. Wood TA, Frenkel EP. An unusual case of macroglobulinemia. Arch Intern Med 1967;119(6):631–7. Available at: https://www.ncbi.nlm.nih.gov/pubmed/4961162.
2. Osterberg G, Rausing A. Reticulum cell sarcoma in Waldenstrom's macroglobulinemia after chlorambucil treatment. Acta Med Scand 1970;188(6):497–504.
3. MacKenzie MR, Fudenberg HH. Macroglobulinemia: an analysis for forty patients. Blood 1972;39(6):874–89. Available at: https://www.ncbi.nlm.nih.gov/pubmed/4623914.
4. Skarin ATL JC. Case records of the Massachusetts General Hospital. Weekly clinicopathological exercises. Case 6-1978. N Engl J Med 1978;298(7):387–96.
5. Choi YJ, Yeh G, Reiner L, et al. Immunoblastic sarcoma following Waldenstrom's macroglobulinemia. Am J Clin Pathol 1979;71(1):121–4.
6. Leonhard SA, Muhleman AF, Hurtubise PE, et al. Emergence of immunoblastic sarcoma in Waldenstrom's macroglobulinemia. Cancer 1980;45(12):3102–7.
7. Garcia R, Hernandez JM, Caballero MD, et al. Immunoblastic lymphoma and associated non-lymphoid malignancies following two cases of Waldenstrom's macroglobulinemia. A review of the literature. Eur J Haematol 1993;50(5): 299–301.
8. Durot E, Tomowiak C, Michallet AS, et al. Transformed Waldenstrom macroglobulinaemia: clinical presentation and outcome. A multi-institutional retrospective study of 77 cases from the French Innovative Leukemia Organization (FILO). Br J Haematol 2017;179(3):439–48.
9. Castillo JJ, Gustine J, Meid K, et al. Histological transformation to diffuse large B-cell lymphoma in patients with Waldenstrom macroglobulinemia. Am J Hematol 2016;91(10):1032–5.
10. Zanwar S, Abeykoon JP, Durot E, et al. Impact of MYD88(L265P) mutation status on histological transformation of Waldenstrom macroglobulinemia. Am J Hematol 2020;95(3):274–81.
11. Durot E, Kanagaratnam L, Zanwar S, et al. A prognostic index predicting survival in transformed Waldenstrom macroglobulinemia. Haematologica 2021;106(11): 2940–6.
12. Treon SP, Gustine J, Xu L, et al. MYD88 wild-type Waldenstrom macroglobulinaemia: differential diagnosis, risk of histological transformation, and overall survival. Br J Haematol 2018;180(3):374–80.
13. Durot E, Kanagaratnam L, Zanwar S, et al. High frequency of central nervous system involvement in transformed Waldenstrom macroglobulinemia. Blood Adv 2022;6(12):3655–8.
14. Leblond V, Johnson S, Chevret S, et al. Results of a randomized trial of chlorambucil versus fludarabine for patients with untreated Waldenstrom macroglobulinemia, marginal zone lymphoma, or lymphoplasmacytic lymphoma. J Clin Oncol 2013;31(3):301–7.
15. Leleu X, Soumerai J, Roccaro A, et al. Increased incidence of transformation and myelodysplasia/acute leukemia in patients with Waldenstrom macroglobulinemia treated with nucleoside analogs. J Clin Oncol 2009;27(2):250–5.
16. Tam CS, Opat S, D'Sa S, et al. A randomized phase 3 trial of zanubrutinib vs ibrutinib in symptomatic Waldenstrom macroglobulinemia: the ASPEN study. Blood 2020;136(18):2038–50.
17. Castillo JJ, Meid K, Gustine JN, et al. Long-term follow-up of ibrutinib monotherapy in treatment-naive patients with Waldenstrom macroglobulinemia. Leukemia 2022;36(2):532–9.

18. Treon SP, Meid K, Gustine J, et al. Long-term follow-up of ibrutinib monotherapy in symptomatic, previously treated patients with Waldenstrom macroglobulinemia. J Clin Oncol 2021;39(6):565–75.
19. Buske C, Tedeschi A, Trotman J, et al. Ibrutinib plus rituximab versus placebo plus rituximab for waldenstrom's macroglobulinemia: final analysis from the randomized phase III iNNOVATE study. J Clin Oncol 2022;40(1):52–62.
20. Hunter ZR, Xu L, Tsakmaklis N, et al. Insights into the genomic landscape of MYD88 wild-type Waldenstrom macroglobulinemia. Blood Adv 2018;2(21):2937–46.
21. Banwait R, Aljawai Y, Cappuccio J, et al. Extramedullary Waldenström macroglobulinemia. Am J Hematol 2015;90(2):100–4.
22. Stien S, Durot E, Durlach A, et al. Cutaneous involvement in Waldenstrom's macroglobulinaemia. Acta Derm Venereol 2020;100(15):adv00225.
23. Alaggio R, Amador C, Anagnostopoulos I, et al. The 5th edition of the World Health Organization classification of haematolymphoid tumours: lymphoid neoplasms. Leukemia 2022;36(7):1720–48.
24. King RL, Goodlad JR, Calaminici M, et al. Lymphomas arising in immune-privileged sites: insights into biology, diagnosis, and pathogenesis. Virchows Arch 2020;476(5):647–65.
25. Mauro FR, Chauvie S, Paoloni F, et al. Diagnostic and prognostic role of PET/CT in patients with chronic lymphocytic leukemia and progressive disease. Leukemia 2015;29(6):1360–5.
26. Banwait R, O'Regan K, Campigotto F, et al. The role of 18F-FDG PET/CT imaging in Waldenstrom macroglobulinemia. Am J Hematol 2011;86(7):567–72.
27. Lin P, Mansoor A, Bueso-Ramos C, et al. Diffuse large B-cell lymphoma occurring in patients with lymphoplasmacytic lymphoma/Waldenstrom macroglobulinemia. Clinicopathologic features of 12 cases. Am J Clin Pathol 2003;120(2):246–53.
28. Owen RG, Bynoe AG, Varghese A, et al. Heterogeneity of histological transformation events in Waldenstrom's macroglobulinemia (WM) and related disorders. Clin Lymphoma Myeloma Leuk 2011;11(1):176–9.
29. Hans CP, Weisenburger DD, Greiner TC, et al. Confirmation of the molecular classification of diffuse large B-cell lymphoma by immunohistochemistry using a tissue microarray. Blood 2004;103(1):275–82.
30. Boiza-Sanchez M, Manso R, Balague O, et al. Lymphoplasmacytic lymphoma associated with diffuse large B-cell lymphoma: progression or divergent evolution? PLoS One 2020;15(11):e0241634.
31. Rossi D, Spina V, Deambrogi C, et al. The genetics of Richter syndrome reveals disease heterogeneity and predicts survival after transformation. Blood 2011;117(12):3391–401 (In eng).
32. Talaulikar D, Biscoe A, Lim JH, et al. Genetic analysis of diffuse large B-cell lymphoma occurring in cases with antecedent Waldenstrom macroglobulinaemia reveals different patterns of clonal evolution. Br J Haematol 2019;185(4):767–70.
33. Jimenez C, Alonso-Alvarez S, Alcoceba M, et al. From Waldenstrom's macroglobulinemia to aggressive diffuse large B-cell lymphoma: a whole-exome analysis of abnormalities leading to transformation. Blood Cancer J 2017;7(8):e591.
34. Tsimberidou AM, O'Brien S, Khouri I, et al. Clinical outcomes and prognostic factors in patients with Richter's syndrome treated with chemotherapy or chemoimmunotherapy with or without stem-cell transplantation. J Clin Oncol 2006;24(15):2343–51.
35. Rusconi C, Anastasia A, Chiarenza A, et al. Outcome of transformed follicular lymphoma worsens according to the timing of transformation and to the number

of previous therapies. A retrospective multicenter study on behalf of Fondazione Italiana Linfomi (FIL). Br J Haematol 2019;185(4):713–7.

36. Link BK, Maurer MJ, Nowakowski GS, et al. Rates and outcomes of follicular lymphoma transformation in the immunochemotherapy era: a report from the University of Iowa/Mayo Clinic Specialized Program of Research Excellence Molecular Epidemiology Resource. J Clin Oncol 2013;31(26):3272–8.

37. Wang Y, Link BK, Witzig TE, et al. Impact of concurrent indolent lymphoma on the clinical outcome of newly diagnosed diffuse large B-cell lymphoma. Blood 2019; 134(16):1289–97.

38. Rovira J, Karube K, Valera A, et al. MYD88 L265P mutations, but no other variants, identify a subpopulation of DLBCL patients of activated B-cell origin, extranodal involvement, and poor outcome. Clin Cancer Res 2016;22(11):2755–64.

39. Vermaat JS, Somers SF, de Wreede LC, et al. MYD88 mutations identify a molecular subgroup of diffuse large B-cell lymphoma with an unfavorable prognosis. Haematologica 2020;105(2):424–34.

40. Villa D, George A, Seymour JF, et al. Favorable outcomes from allogeneic and autologous stem cell transplantation for patients with transformed nonfollicular indolent lymphoma. Biol Blood Marrow Transplant 2014;20(11):1813–8.

41. Blaker YN, Eide MB, Liestol K, et al. High dose chemotherapy with autologous stem cell transplant for patients with transformed B-cell non-Hodgkin lymphoma in the rituximab era. Leuk Lymphoma 2014;55(10):2319–27.

42. Villa D, Crump M, Keating A, et al. Outcome of patients with transformed indolent non-Hodgkin lymphoma referred for autologous stem-cell transplantation. Ann Oncol 2013;24(6):1603–9.

43. Ban-Hoefen M, Vanderplas A, Crosby-Thompson AL, et al. Transformed non-Hodgkin lymphoma in the rituximab era: analysis of the NCCN outcomes database. Br J Haematol 2013;163(4):487–95.

44. Madsen C, Pedersen MB, Vase MO, et al. Outcome determinants for transformed indolent lymphomas treated with or without autologous stem-cell transplantation. Ann Oncol 2015;26(2):393–9.

45. Kuruvilla J, MacDonald DA, Kouroukis CT, et al. Salvage chemotherapy and autologous stem cell transplantation for transformed indolent lymphoma: a subset analysis of NCIC CTG LY12. Blood 2015;126(6):733–8.

46. Chin CK, Lim KJ, Lewis K, et al. Autologous stem cell transplantation for untreated transformed indolent B-cell lymphoma in first remission: an international, multi-centre propensity-score-matched study. Br J Haematol 2020;191(5): 806–15.

47. Schmitz N, Zeynalova S, Nickelsen M, et al. CNS international prognostic index: a risk model for CNS relapse in patients with diffuse large B-cell lymphoma treated with R-CHOP. J Clin Oncol 2016;34(26):3150–6.

48. Villa D, Connors JM, Shenkier TN, et al. Incidence and risk factors for central nervous system relapse in patients with diffuse large B-cell lymphoma: the impact of the addition of rituximab to CHOP chemotherapy. Ann Oncol 2010;21(5): 1046–52.

49. El-Galaly TC, Cheah CY, Bendtsen MD, et al. Treatment strategies, outcomes and prognostic factors in 291 patients with secondary CNS involvement by diffuse large B-cell lymphoma. Eur J Cancer 2018;93:57–68.

50. Eyre TA, Djebbari F, Kirkwood AA, et al. Efficacy of central nervous system prophylaxis with stand-alone intrathecal chemotherapy in diffuse large B-cell lymphoma patients treated with anthracycline-based chemotherapy in the rituximab era: a systematic review. Haematologica 2020;105(7):1914–24.

51. Orellana-Noia VM, Reed DR, McCook AA, et al. Single-route CNS prophylaxis for aggressive non-Hodgkin lymphomas: real-world outcomes from 21 US academic institutions. Blood 2022;139(3):413–23.
52. Puckrin R, El Darsa H, Ghosh S, et al. Ineffectiveness of high-dose methotrexate for prevention of CNS relapse in diffuse large B-cell lymphoma. Am J Hematol 2021;96(7):764–71.
53. Fleming M, Huang Y, Dotson E, et al. Feasibility of high-dose methotrexate administered on day 1 of (R)CHOP in aggressive non-Hodgkin lymphomas. Blood Adv 2022;6(2):460–72.
54. Wilson MR, Eyre TA, Kirkwood AA, et al. Timing of high-dose methotrexate CNS prophylaxis in DLBCL: a multicenter international analysis of 1384 patients. Blood 2022;139(16):2499–511.
55. Castillo JJ, Allan JN, Siddiqi T, et al. Venetoclax in previously treated waldenstrom macroglobulinemia. J Clin Oncol 2022;40(1):63–71.
56. Younes A, Sehn LH, Johnson P, et al. Randomized PHASE III trial of ibrutinib and rituximab plus cyclophosphamide, doxorubicin, vincristine, and prednisone in non-germinal center B-cell diffuse large B-cell lymphoma. J Clin Oncol 2019; 37(15):1285–95.
57. Morschhauser F, Feugier P, Flinn IW, et al. A phase 2 study of venetoclax plus R-CHOP as first-line treatment for patients with diffuse large B-cell lymphoma. Blood 2021;137(5):600–9.
58. Neelapu SS, Locke FL, Bartlett NL, et al. Axicabtagene ciloleucel CAR T-cell therapy in refractory large B-cell lymphoma. N Engl J Med 2017;377(26):2531–44.
59. Schuster SJ, Bishop MR, Tam CS, et al. Tisagenlecleucel in adult relapsed or refractory diffuse large B-cell lymphoma. N Engl J Med 2019;380(1):45–56.
60. Locke FL, Miklos DB, Jacobson CA, et al. Axicabtagene ciloleucel as second-line therapy for large B-cell lymphoma. N Engl J Med 2022;386(7):640–54.
61. Bishop MR, Dickinson M, Purtill D, et al. Second-line tisagenlecleucel or standard care in aggressive B-cell lymphoma. N Engl J Med 2022;386(7):629–39.
62. Palomba ML, Qualls D, Monette S, et al. CD19-directed chimeric antigen receptor T cell therapy in Waldenstrom macroglobulinemia: a preclinical model and initial clinical experience. J Immunother Cancer 2022;10(2). https://doi.org/10.1136/jitc-2021-004128.
63. Abramson JS, Palomba ML, Gordon LI, et al. Lisocabtagene maraleucel for patients with relapsed or refractory large B-cell lymphomas (TRANSCEND NHL 001): a multicentre seamless design study. Lancet 2020;396(10254):839–52.
64. Bansal R, Jurcic JG, Sawas A, et al. Chimeric antigen receptor T cells for treatment of transformed Waldenstrom macroglobulinemia. Leuk Lymphoma 2020; 61(2):465–8.
65. Durot E, Tomowiak C, Toussaint E, et al. Transformed waldenstrom macroglobulinemia: update on diagnosis, prognosis and treatment. Hemato 2022;3(4): 650–62. Available at: https://www.mdpi.com/2673-6357/3/4/44.

Management of Waldenström Macroglobulinemia in Limited-Resource Settings

Eloisa Riva, MD[a], Vania Tietsche de Moraes Hungría, MD[b],
Carlos Chiattone, MD[c], Humberto Martínez-Cordero, MD, MSc[d],*

KEYWORDS

- Waldenström macroglobulinemia • Immunohistochemistry (IHC) • IgM-MGUS
- Lymphoplasmacytic lymphoma

KEY POINTS

- The diagnosis and management of Waldenstrom's Macroglobulinemia (WM) in low-income areas may be more difficult than in developed countries.
- Lack of access to diagnostic and treatment technologies in regions with limited resources is the general rule.
- Local studies found a 5-year OS rate of 81%, showing comparable results with other latitudes.
- Chemoimmunotherapy with dexamethasone, rituximab, and cyclophosphamide is the most common first-line treatment.
- Here we suggest solutions to address disparities in treatment, such as promoting specialized units and increasing access to clinical trials.

INTRODUCTION

Waldenström macroglobulinemia (WM) is a rare, highly heterogeneous, and incurable B-cell malignancy classified as a monoclonal gammopathy that, unlike multiple myeloma, is more common in Caucasians than in African descent.[1,2] Epidemiology is known in countries such as the United States and Europe, where the incidence, prevalence, and mortality have been described.[3,4] However, more data are needed from regions with limited resources. In Latin America and Asia, studies on the disease

[a] Clinical Hospital Dr Manuel Quintela, University of the Republic, British Hospital, Montevideo, Uruguay; [b] Irmandade Da Santa Casa De Misericordia De São Paulo, Sao Paulo, Brazil; [c] Hematology and Oncology Discipline, Santa Casa Medical School, Sao Paulo, Brazil; [d] Insituto Nacional de Cancerología, Bogotá, Colombia and Hospital Militar Central de Colombia
* Corresponding author. Calle 1 No 9-85 Bogotá, Colombia.
E-mail addresses: rmartinez@cancer.gov.co; humbertomartinez48@hotmail.com

Hematol Oncol Clin N Am 37 (2023) 801–807
https://doi.org/10.1016/j.hoc.2023.04.010
0889-8588/23/© 2023 Elsevier Inc. All rights reserved.

denote essential aspects such as clinical behavior, treatment patterns, and prognosis.[5,6] During the past 2 decades, advances in the condition have been crucial but unfortunately diagnostic and treatment technologies are rarely available in some resource-limited regions.[5–7] This article aims to address the essential aspects of WM in low-income areas in terms of the epidemiology of the disease, access to drugs and prognosis, as well as to develop adapted recommendations, including some possible alternatives regarding diagnosis and treatment.

METHODS

A writing group of physicians with experience in the care of WM in Latin America was convened to redact this document. First, we performed a PubMed and gray literature search using the terms "Waldenström macroglobulinemia," "non-Hodgkin lymphoma," "low income," "limited resources," and "Latin America." We focused on general epidemiology, diagnosis, staging, risk assessment, and management. In the end, we made some recommendations based on the available published evidence and personal experience (expert opinion), with consensus among the writing group members if a higher level of evidence was unavailable.

EPIDEMIOLOGY OF WALDENSTRÖM MACROGLOBULINEMIA

WM is a rare disease, with a reported incidence of approximately 3 to 4 cases per million per year, increasing with age to 30 per million at 80 years. It represents 3% of all monoclonal gammopathies (17% of immunoglobulin M [IgM] gammopathies) and 2% of lymphomas.[1,2] The incidence and mortality differ significantly by geographic location, race, age, sex, the primary site of involvement, and subtype between resource-limited regions and North American countries.[2,3] A Korean study of newly diagnosed patients with WM found the incidence to be 0.10 per year in 2016, and the prevalence was 0.42 per 100.000 person-years in the same year. They found a standardized mortality ratio of 7.57.[6] One population-based study was performed in China, where 4472 patients were included from 9 The Surveillance, Epidemiology, and End Results (SEER) registries from 1980 to 2016; they found a global incidence and mortality of 0.48 and 0.34 per 100,000 person-years, respectively.[8]

WM is more frequent in men with a male-to-female of 3 to 1, and the survival decreases as age increases; however, some studies have found a dramatic increase in the 5-year survival rate from the 1980s to 2010s (48 vs 69%).[8]

The first Latin American study to provide real-world data on WM has been recently published. In this retrospective analysis, 159 patients with WM were included in the local WM registries in 24 centers from 7 countries between 1991 and 2019. The median age at diagnosis was 67 years, and 62% were male with a median follow-up of 69 months; the 5-year overall survival (OS) rate was 81%, which is higher than that found in other latitudes.[5]

DIAGNOSIS, STAGING, AND RISK ASSESSMENT

As per international guidelines, the diagnosis of WM is established when histopathological infiltration by lymphoplasmacytic cells/lymphoplasmacytic lymphoma (LPL) of the bone marrow (BM) is confirmed and the detection of any amount of monoclonal IgM protein, which should always be confirmed by immunofixation. Approximately 90% of patients with WM harbor a somatic mutation in MYD88.[9] Notably, MYD88 mutations have been detected in precursor stages of WM known as IgM monoclonal gammopathy of uncertain significance (IgM-MGUS). They have been associated with a more significant progression from asymptomatic to symptomatic WM and a higher response to Bruton Tirosine Kinase (BTK) inhibitors. One Latin American study performed on 32 patients detected an MYD88 mutation in 20 out of 21 patients with WM (95%), in 1 out of 3 cases of IgM-MGUS (33%), in 1 out of 5 patients with splenic marginal zone lymphoma (SMZL) (20%) and not found in isolated cases of IgG-Lymphoplasmacytic lymphoma (IgG-LPL) (0%), IgM Lymphoplasmacytic lymphoma (IgM-MM) (0%), and Non- cetrogerminal Diffuse Large B cell Lymphoma (DLBCL non-GC) (0%).[10]

The recommended workup should include a complete clinical history, physical examination, and family history of WM and other B-cell lymphoproliferative disorders. The review of systems involves identifying B symptoms, organomegaly, hyperviscosity symptoms, neuropathy, Raynaud disease, rash, peripheral edema, skin abnormalities, dyspnea, and fundoscopic examination.[9] One Mexican study, published in 2015, looking at causes of hyperviscosity syndrome, found the leading causes of the syndrome were multiple myeloma followed by WM and Sjögren disease. The predominant clinical manifestations were neurologic and hemorrhagic symptoms. The highest serum viscosity mean was present in WM and Sjogren syndrome (SS).[11]

The minimal laboratory studies include a complete blood count, serum immunoglobulin levels (IgA, IgG, IgM), serum and urine electrophoresis with immunofixation, metabolic panel, serum B2 microglobulin level, viral serology (hepatitis B virus [HBV], hepatitis C virus [HCV], and human immunodeficiency virus [HIV]), testing for MYD88 L265P mutation, and BM aspiration and biopsy with immunohistochemistry (IHC), which is necessary for the diagnosis. Flow cytometry is an alternative if IHC is not available. If clinically indicated, computed tomography (CT) of the chest, abdomen, and pelvis, cryoglobulins, cold agglutinin titer, serum viscosity, screening for acquired von Willebrand disease, 24-hour urine protein quantification, serum Free Light chains (FLCs), N termina pro B natriuretic peptide (NTproBNP), cardiac troponins, Electromyography (EMG), anti myelin-associated glycoprotein (anti-MAG), Anti-Ganglioside M1 Antibody (anti-GM1), and consultation with neurologist must be requested. Risk factors considered in international prognostic scoring system for Waldenstrom macroglobulinemia (IPSSWM) include are age greater than 65 years, Hb less than 11.5 g/dL, platelets less than 100 × 10^9/L, B2M greater than 3 mg/L, and IgM greater than 70 g/L. Other risk factors not included in IPSSWM include elevated serum LDH and low serum albumin.[9,10]

In the Latin-American study, most patients were symptomatic at diagnosis (95%), probably reflecting delayed access to specialized cancer care. The most common symptoms were symptomatic adenopathy (28%), symptomatic splenomegaly (25%), and hyperviscosity symptoms (20%). B symptoms were present in 18%, symptomatic hepatomegaly present in 13%, peripheral neuropathy present in 11%, and bleeding in only 3% of the patients.[5]

Overall, molecular testing was performed in only 21% of patients. MYD88 L265P testing was performed in 17% (n = 27 of 159), del 17p in 6% (n = 9 of 159), and CXCR4 in 1% (n = 1 of 159) reflecting the lack of generalized access to these tools. For those in whom genetic testing was performed, 89% (n = 24 of 27) had MYD88 L265P mutation, none had del17p mutation, and the only patient tested for CXCR4 mutation had MYD88 L265P and CXCR4 mutations.[5]

One of the first articles published in patients treated with chlorambucil as a monotherapy showed that some pretreatment parameters, including older age, male sex, general symptoms, and cytopenia, carry a poor prognosis in WM. By contrast, high initial tumor burden (indicated by organomegaly, high IgM level, and a high percentage of marrow lymphoid cells) did not seem to be significantly associated with short survival.[12]

When evaluating the risk in the Riva and colleagues study, the IPSSWM score was available in 141 patients, of whom 40%, 37%, and 23% were classified as high-risk, intermediate-risk, and low-risk diseases, respectively.[5]

MANAGEMENT

Recommendations for the initiation of therapy in patients with WM include the presence of fever, which usually is recurrent, night-drenching sweats, significant weight loss, fatigue, hyperviscosity, bulky lymphadenopathy, symptomatic hepatomegaly, or splenomegaly, symptomatic organomegaly and organ or tissue infiltration, and peripheral neuropathy due to WM.[7,9]

Laboratory indications for the initiation of therapy include symptomatic cryoglobulinemia, cold agglutinin anemia, autoimmune hemolytic anemia or thrombocytopenia less than 100×10^9/L, and nephropathy, which must be associated to WM, amyloidosis-related to WM, anemia with Hb lower less than 10 g/dL, and IgM levels greater than 60 g/L.[7,9]

As mentioned above, most of the patients in the Latin-American study were symptomatic at diagnosis; consequently, they all received frontline treatment.[5]

Clinical or laboratory criteria should orient the treatment of WM. The most important aspects are the presence of hyperviscosity, cytopenia, bulky disease, the need for immediate tumor reduction, neuropathy, and WM-related AL amyloidosis.[7,9]

The management of WM is very heterogeneous in low-income countries. Eighty-nine percent of the patients in the registry received treatment, with chemoimmunotherapy in 66% and monotherapy in 25%. The most frequent regimen was dexamethasone, rituximab, and cyclophosphamide. Less than 10% of patients received ibrutinib or bortezomib frontline, probably reflecting the need for more access to these drugs. The most frequent second-line regimens were Bendamustine plus rituximab (BR) and ibrutinib.[5]

The overall response rate to frontline treatment in the Riva and colleagues study was 83%, with the majority achieving only partial response at 53%, and with a median follow-up of 69 months, the 5-year OS rate was 81%. High-risk IPSSWM at treatment initiation was an independent risk factor for OS ($P = .003$) and progression free survival (PFS) ($P = .005$). Worse 5-year OS ($P = .003$) and PFS ($P = .004$) rates were seen in patients with a high-risk IPSSWM score (OS: 64%; PFS: 35%) compared with patients with intermediate-risk (OS: 88%; PFS: 59%) and low-risk (OS: 100%; PFS: 82%) diseases. Men had worse 5-year OS (75% vs 94%, $P = .006$) and PFS (50% vs 72%, $P = .004$) rates than women.[5] **Table 1** shows available treatments in Latin America.

FINAL RECOMMENDATIONS OF THE EXPERT PANEL
Diagnosis

- A complete diagnosis of WM requires confirmation by histopathology demonstrating the BM infiltration by monoclonal lymphoplasmacytic cells typically positive for CD19, CD20, CD22, and CD79a, and serum monoclonal IgM of any amount, confirmed by immunoglobulin M quantitation, serum protein electrophoresis (SPEP), and immunofixation.
- The study of MYD88 L265P mutation is recommended and may help differentiate WM from other lymphoma subtypes such as marginal or IgM multiple myeloma.

Staging and Risk Assessment

- Initial evaluation includes a complete blood cell count, serum biochemistry, B2 microglobulin, serum protein electrophoresis, and IgM quantification.

Table 1
Treatments available in Latin America

Country/Drug Regimen	Ibrutinib	Acalabrutinib	Zanubrutinib	Bendamustine	Rituximab	Bortezomib	ASCT
Colombia							
Brazil							
Uruguay							
Argentina							
Ecuador							
Chile							
Mexico							
Paraguay							
Bolivia							
Venezuela							
Costa Rica							
Guatemala							
Peru							
Panama							
Dominican Republic							

Green: Full access; Yellow: partial access (IE private insurance); Red: no access; Blue: available but with other indications (ie, chronic lymphocytic leukemia or trials); White: no information available.

- Coombs test, cold agglutinins, cryoglobulins, hemolysis tests, and iron status should be done in patients with anemia.
- Consultation with a neurologist is recommended in patients with neuropathy.
- A funduscopic examination and ophthalmology consultation are highly recommended in patients with suspected hyperviscosity syndrome.
- Fat abdomen aspirate stained with Congo red and cardiac and renal biomarkers should be done in patients with suspected amyloidosis.
- Contrast-enhanced CT is highly recommended as an initial imaging study to detect nodal component.
- The IPSSWM is recommended to define high-risk patients.

Management

- Asymptomatic patients should not be treated and continue to follow up every 3 to 6 months.
- Plasmapheresis should be used with appropriate systemic therapy in patients with hyperviscosity in an emergency.
- Therapy is indicated in case of drenching sweating, unexplained fever, significant weight loss, cytopenia, hyperviscosity, moderate neuropathy, WM-associated systemic amyloidosis, cryoglobulinemia, or cold agglutinin disease.
- Combinations of rituximab with alkylating agents (oral or I.V. cyclophosphamide, bendamustine, or chlorambucil) or proteasome inhibitors are recommended as initial treatment options.
- Single-agent therapy with alkylating agents or nucleoside analogs or rituximab should be considered for frail patients or unfit for more effective chemoimmunotherapy combinations.
- Maintenance treatment with rituximab is not recommended for patients with WM.
- For patients who have relapsed within 12 months from chemoimmunotherapy, including rituximab-refractory patients, single-agent ibrutinib should always be considered as second-line treatment.
- For patients ineligible for chemoimmunotherapy at first-line, single-agent ibrutinib may be considered.
- For patients with late relapses after chemoimmunotherapy, retreatment with chemoimmunotherapy could be an option; however, ibrutinib may be considered.
- High-dose therapy with autologous hematopoietic cell transplantation may be considered in selected young patients with chemo-sensitive relapse, considering its availability in most low-income countries.
- Although participation in clinical trials is strongly encouraged for some patients in the first or subsequent lines of therapy, this possibility is not always available in low-income countries. Expert consultation is recommended in this scenario.

Disparities and Approach to a Solution

To overcome the disparities in treatment, the involvement of various actors is required, such as regional experts, government authorities, and cancer reference centers, to promote specialized units in the management of this disease, achieve greater participation in clinical trials, increase local research, as well as have access to proven effective technologies in the diagnosis and management of this disease.

CLINICS CARE POINTS

- Early diagnosis and risk stratification is essential to improve outcomes in Waldenstrom's Macroglobulinemia.

- Asymptomatic patients should not be treated however the follow-up is vital.
- Several treatment are available to treat patients with Waldentrom's Macroglobulinemia frequently not available in Latin America.
- To overcome disparities in Waldenstrom's Macroglobulinemia various specialists are required to work together with the aim to create specialized units, achieve greater participation in clinical traials and increase local research.

ACKNOWLEDGEMENT

The authors would like to thank Dr Jorge Castillo for improving the content of this documment. We did not have financial support.

REFERENCES

1. García-Sanz R, Montoto S, Torrequebrada A, et al. Waldenström macroglobulinaemia: Presenting features and outcome in a series with 217 cases. Br J Haematol 2001;115(3):575–82.
2. Wang H, Chen Y, Li F, et al. Temporal and geographic variations of Waldenstrom macroglobulinemia incidence: A large population-based study. Cancer 2012; 118(15):3793–800.
3. Castillo JJ, Olszewski AJ, Kanan S, et al. Overall survival and competing risks of death in patients with Waldenström macroglobulinaemia: An analysis of the Surveillance, Epidemiology and End Results database. Br J Haematol 2015;169(1):81–9.
4. Pophali PA, Bartley A, Kapoor P, et al. Prevalence and survival of smouldering Waldenström macroglobulinaemia in the United States. Br J Haematol 2019; 184(6):1014–7.
5. Riva E, Duarte PJ, Valcárcel B, et al. Treatment and Survival Outcomes of Waldenstrom Macroglobulinemia in Latin American Patients: A Multinational Retrospective Cohort Study. JCO Glob Oncol 2022;(8):1–12.
6. Jeong S, Kong SG, Kim DJ, et al. Incidence, prevalence, mortality, and causes of death in Waldenström macroglobulinemia: A nationwide, population-based cohort study. BMC Cancer 2020;20(1):1–9.
7. Castillo JJ, Advani RH, Branagan AR, et al. Consensus treatment recommendations from the tenth International Workshop for Waldenström Macroglobulinaemia. Lancet Haematol 2020;7(11):e827–37.
8. Yin X, Chen L, Fan F, et al. Trends in Incidence and Mortality of Waldenström Macroglobulinemia: A Population-Based Study. Front Oncol 2020;10:1712 [Erratum in: Front Oncol. 2021 Feb 18;11:657016. PMID: 33014849; PMCID: PMC7511580].
9. Staber PB, Kersten MJ. EHA Endorsement of ESMO Clinical Practice Guidelines for Diagnosis, Treatment, and Follow-up for Waldenström's Macroglobulinemia. Hemasphere 2021;5(10):e634.
10. Giuliani F, Pavlovsky MA, Giere I, et al. First Latin America report on the diagnostic utility of the study of the MYD88 L265P gene mutation in patients with Waldenström Macroglobulinemia. Ann Hematol 2022;101(10):2365–7.
11. Armillas-Canseco F, Martinez-Baños D, Hernandez-Mata C, et al. Hyperviscosity Syndrome: A 30-year Experience in a Reference Center in Mexico City. Abstract| 2017;17(supplement 2):s342.
12. Facon T, Brouillard M, Duhamel A, et al. Prognostic factors in Waldenström's macroglobulinemia: a report of 167 cases. J Clin Oncol 1993;11(8):1553–8.

Moving?

Make sure your subscription moves with you!

To notify us of your new address, find your **Clinics Account Number** (located on your mailing label above your name), and contact customer service at:

Email: **journalscustomerservice-usa@elsevier.com**

800-654-2452 (subscribers in the U.S. & Canada)
314-447-8871 (subscribers outside of the U.S. & Canada)

Fax number: **314-447-8029**

Elsevier Health Sciences Division
Subscription Customer Service
3251 Riverport Lane
Maryland Heights, MO 63043

*To ensure uninterrupted delivery of your subscription, please notify us at least 4 weeks in advance of move.